KU-165-598

How not to be a doctor

and other essays

How not to be a doctor
and other essays

John Launer
**Tavistock Clinic, London
and
London Department of Postgraduate
Medical Education**

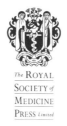

The ROYAL
SOCIETY of
MEDICINE
PRESS Limited

© 2007 John Launer

These articles were originally published in QJM between 2002 and 2006, reprinted with permission of the publisher

Published by the Royal Society of Medicine Press Ltd
1 Wimpole Street, London W1G 0AE, UK
Tel: +44 (0)20 7290 2921
Fax: +44 (0)20 7290 2929
E-mail: publishing@rsm.ac.uk
Website: www.rsmpress.co.uk

Apart from any fair dealing for the purposes of research or private study, criticism or review, as permitted under the UK Copyright, Designs and Patents Act, 1988, no part of this publication may be reproduced, stored or transmitted, in any form or by any means, without the prior permission in writing of the publishers or in the case of reprographic reproduction in accordance with the terms of licences issued by the Copyright Licensing Agency in the UK, or in accordance with the terms of licences issued by the appropriate Reproduction Rights Organization outside the UK. Enquiries concerning reproduction outside the terms stated here should be sent to the publishers at the UK address printed on this page.

The right of John Launer to be identified as author of this work has been asserted by him in accordance with the Copyright, Designs and Patents Act, 1988.

British Library Cataloguing in Publication Data
A catalogue record for this book is available from the British Library

ISBN 978-1-85315-752-3

Distribution in Europe and Rest of World:

Marston Book Services Ltd
PO Box 269
Abingdon
Oxon OX14 4YN, UK
Tel: +44 (0)1235 465500
Fax: +44 (0)1235 465555
Email: direct.order@marston.co.uk

Distribution in the USA and Canada:
Royal Society of Medicine Press Ltd
c/o BookMasters, Inc.
30 Amberwood Parkway
Ashland, Ohio 44805, USA
Tel: +1 800 247 6553/ +1 800 266 5564
Fax: +1 419 281 6883
Email: order@bookmasters.com

Distribution in Australia and New Zealand:
Elsevier Australia
30-52 Smidmore Street
Marrickville NSW 2204, Australia
Tel: +61 2 9349 5811
Fax: +61 2 9349 5911
Email: service@elsevier.com.au

Typeset by Saxon Graphics, Derby, UK

Printed and bound by Krips, The Netherlands

Contents

Foreword

by Christopher Martyn

Sir Thomas Beecham, the celebrated conductor, was uncompromising in expecting his audiences to engage with new compositions by living composers. But, after the main part of the concert was over, he was not above rewarding them with something short, lively and easy to listen to. These pieces famously became known as Beecham lollipops. When I was the editor of the *QJM*, it occurred to me that its readers deserved something similar. I thought that after grappling with the serious scientific stuff, they might like to read something intended to give pleasure rather than instruction.

So I asked John Launer if he would be prepared to write a regular column to appear at the end of each issue. I made no stipulation about the subjects that he should tackle, and none about the style in which he should write. The only thing I suggested was that he should bear in mind that the core readership of the journal consisted mainly of fairly senior and fairly academic physicians. He understood at once what I was getting at: while he could say what he pleased, write to annoy or delight whomever he liked, he need not pull his punches. This was a readership that thought for themselves and could take it on the chin.

Every month for five years, John produced a column, which appeared under the title *Coda* at the end of each issue. They were usually reflections, in one way or another, on the art, practice or teaching of medicine. Their range was astonishing: sometimes self-mocking (The Wrong Trousers); now and again subversive (Careers Advice); often moving (Seeing Double); occasionally erudite (Mysteries of the Male); but always ironic and humane. They rapidly developed a cult following. People would tell me that they cut them out to pin on their departmental notice board. Minerva's column in the *BMJ* often picked them up for comment. On *QJM's* website, they received more hits than many of the scientific papers. I'm delighted that the Royal Society of Medicine Press has now made them available to a wider audience.

Whoever dubbed the pieces that Beecham played at the end of his concerts 'lollipops' was being unfair. They weren't sugary confections without nutritious value but brief pieces of good music. And when I used the same metaphor about John's essays, I was making a similar mistake. Certainly, they are easy to read, but that's because he writes so well. Yet there's an underlying, if lightly worn, seriousness of purpose. His intent is always to stimulate his readers to question their certainties and to challenge the orthodox. But why do I waste your time by trying to describe them? Turn the page and enjoy.

Author's Note

Some of the essays in this book include stories about patients. In every case I have changed personal details, or combined several different encounters, so that no-one could be identified.

While writing these pieces, I nearly always received helpful comments from family, colleagues and friends. I particularly want to acknowledge the steadfast support of Dr Christopher Martyn, my wife Rabbi Lee Wax, and the late Dr Brian Snowdon. This collection is dedicated in memory of Brian.

1 Stress test

The ECG technician came out of her room and bellowed a name at us: 'Andrew Parkinson!'. There was silence, as we all looked at each other sheepishly. Apart from myself, all the other people sitting in the queue were elderly women, some of them from the wards, and wearing dressing gowns. 'Andrew Parkinson!!' she shouted again, this time fixing me with an accusatory look. 'John Launer?' I said guiltily. She looked again at the form in her hand. 'Bloody hell,' she said, 'I've already done Andrew Parkinson.' She disappeared, and came back a minute later with another form. 'John Launer!' she bellowed this time, as if I might have changed my identity in the meantime.

I went into the ECG room and she told me to strip to the waist, and that she was going to shave some small areas on my chest. No introduction, no preliminaries, no questions, no explanations, no friendly chatter to put me at my ease. 'Get up on the treadmill ... I'm going to stick some pads on your chest ... JESUS!' She had just seen my initial tracing. Immediately, she tore off a length of it and scurried off without another word. I could hear her anxious conversation with the junior doctor on the other side of the curtain. I wasn't very surprised when she came back to ask me if I had ever had an ECG before. It was still an odd question. Is anyone ever sent for a stress test without first having a resting ECG? Besides, my notes were in front of her, stuffed with previous ECGs. 'Yes', I answered. 'I've got left bundle branch block. I've always had it.' I wondered for an instant if it was worth expressing my doubts that the stress test was likely to be very reliable anyway, given my abnormality, but I thought better of it. The appointment had come as part of a package of tests before I could see the cardiologist again, and I had already resolved to surrender to the machine, both literally and figuratively.

Incurious about my use of the technical term, she scurried away once more for another half-whispered conversation behind the curtain, and then returned, apparently reassured. 'I'm a doctor', I added – mainly to satisfy an inner need. I certainly had little expectation that it would lead to a change in her manner. She started to press buttons, and the treadmill gathered speed each time. After a while I asked her if it was OK to run, as I was accustomed to jogging and found it more comfortable than having to walk very fast. She said I could, but a few minutes later she commented how much I was perspiring, especially for someone who was used to jogging. It was a very hot day, and there wasn't a fan in the room. I refrained from pointing out that someone coming for a stress ECG to find out if they possibly needed heart surgery might, just conceivably, be perspiring from anxiety, even without a technician whose gift for empathy was small.

As I reached stage 5 on the Bruce protocol, she told me that my shoulders seemed unusually tense. This was interfering with the tracing, and anyway they shouldn't be like that if I exercised regularly. I asked her how much faster the treadmill would go, and she told me there wasn't a limit. She then waited another couple of minutes before giving me the information I obviously wanted, namely whether she would stop before I got exhausted. Finally, she did turn the treadmill off and I could see (by squinting sideways) that my pulse rate had reached 180 without any obvious sign of ischaemia – for what that was worth. I asked her if I was right in thinking the tracing looked pretty fine. 'Which consultant are you under?' was her response. I gave his name. 'He'll tell you at your next appointment. Here's a towel for the sweat. You can put on your clothes now, we're finished.' A few weeks later I had the test I really needed - a stress echocardiogram - which was normal.

The experience was excruciating, a needless act of emotional abuse where kindness would have required little effort. It was also, I suppose, no more and no less cruel than thousands of such encounters that occur every day in the health service, not just with technicians, but with doctors, clerks, or just about anyone with a degree of power to exercise and who lacks insight – whether for a passing moment or a whole lifetime – into what it feels like to be the other. We all have our explanations for such behaviour. They include multiple failings at the collective level: in the department, the hospital, the health service, and the nation. We also have our own preferred prescriptions for the problem, such as better pay and conditions, improved team morale, enhanced training, attractive incentives, consumer choice, becoming a more compassionate society, and so on and so forth.

The philosopher Martin Buber taught that we all live with a two-fold attitude, which he called the 'I-It' attitude and the 'I-Thou' attitude. '*If I face a human being as my Thou*' he argued, '*he is not a thing among things, and does not consist of things*'. In the same corridor as the ECG technician, there is a secretary who is outstandingly helpful, although presumably she shares many of the same work conditions as the technician. I know her name, her direct line and her email address. She always remembers my name, what I do, who I am seeing and why. When I contact her, she seems to operate from the premise that my request is going to be reasonable and that she will try her utmost to make sure it is met. I believe she treats everyone else in the same way. Without the active will, and the moral choice, of people like her, I suspect that all the well-meant interventions of politicians, managers and educators to improve the way patients are treated will subside into mere noise. Or to put it in Buber's words: '*All true living is meeting.*'

2 Of cheese and choice

I am standing by the cheese cabinet in our local supermarket. (This is poetic licence, you understand. I am actually sitting at my PC, but my recent supermarket experience is so vivid that I have no difficulty reliving it.) I am in a state of high anxiety. In front of me are uncountable types of cheese. There is Canadian, Irish, Welsh, New Zealand and English. There is mild, mature, extra-mature, vintage and farmhouse. There is low fat, full fat – presumably 'high fat' would be a marketing disaster – and vegetarian. There are special cheeses in expensive waxy paper, or in the kind of customized black rind you see in Dutch markets. There is also 'value' cheese with a naff logo that allows you to proclaim your penury or your meanness. These are the varieties of Cheddar alone.

Faced with such an obscene superfluity of Cheddars, how can I be certain of selecting the best value, the best taste, or exactly the one my wife will like? Being of a moderately obsessional turn of mind, I try to contain my anxiety by doing a mathematical calculation of how many different options there must be here: nationality times maturity, maturity times fat content, fat content times price band, and so on. The arithmetic soon falters. Firstly, it is clear that the grid may have gaps in it (the Welsh seem to make mature vegetarian Cheddar, but the Irish do not). I also start to have serious doubts as to whether I fully understand the taxonomy of Cheddar: is there such a thing as a mild farmhouse or an extra-mature non-vintage? I even begin to wonder if I shall need to invoke Venn diagrams or algorithms to sort the problem out.

Then something else occurs to me. The cheeses are not laid out systematically. Their arrangement is apparently haphazard. Low fat Irish Cheddar jostles alongside Olde Mother Bassington's Superior Special Original Connoisseur Edition from the Cheddar Gorge, but nowhere near any of its creamier compatriots. Expensive cheeses are mixed promiscuously with the cheapos. If you are searching for a mild English vegetarian cheese – and suddenly I remember that is exactly what my wife asked for – you may need to scrutinize the contents of this cabinet for hours.

Finally, the penny drops. There is method in this madness. I am being intentionally bamboozled. The proprietors of this supermarket do not want me to make a rational choice. Quite the contrary. The ridiculous volume of information, the gratuitous scale of alternatives, and the brazen attack on my cognitive ability are all calculated to render me incapable of choice. As a result, I will almost certainly end up choosing a cheese impulsively and at random. I will be left, of course, with the feeling that I could have chosen better. Like a teasing lover, the supermarket has promised me all, but will deliver so little that I will surely be coming back for more.

Having got a handle on this, I find that my mind starts to wander to another topic: choice in health care. Perhaps this is not surprising. The issue of choice for patients has acquired stupendous prominence in British political discourse. We can now choose from as wide a variety of hospitals and consultants as we can with cheeses. Both the main political parties are also promising, in different ways, to extend even further the choices that are open to patients. Both are proclaiming that choice is the route to patient autonomy, to increased consumer influence, and therefore to raised standards.

At one level, this is entirely welcome. Twenty years ago, I was able to make a referral as a GP to any specialist in the country, but successive reorganizations of the health service (some of them, oddly enough, in the name of competition) reduced my options drastically. It is nice that I will be able to choose again. However, the example of the cheese cabinet may indicate what happens when choice alone is king. What I most longed for when I stood by the cheese counter was for a friend to appear unexpectedly from around the corner to say: 'Go for the own-brand farmhouse, John. It's fantastic!' In much the same spirit, our patients often ask us: 'What would *you* recommend?' or 'What would you do if you were in my shoes?' These questions might appear like passivity, or as attempts to evoke paternalism, but usually they are not. They are forms of acknowledgement that what raises our fear are the unknown and the overwhelming, and what allays it are trust and human connectedness.

There is, in fact, a certain cynicism about placing such an emphasis on choice. In the real world, as opposed to the virtual one that politicians so often seem to inhabit, many of the neediest people cannot actually exercise very much choice in these matters for all sort of reasons: infirmity, urgency, distance from other providers, the complexity of their needs, or the natural wish to be near their families. But even for the small proportion of patients who are wealthy and well enough to travel anywhere for their medical care, choice may not be so very liberating either. Giving them a list of the nearest eight hospitals, together with records on surgical mortality, cross-infection and a vast array of other parameters may only raise their anxiety – for who can ever be sure that they could not have had their gall bladder or cataract removed just a little more slickly, a little more painlessly, somewhere else? Like the bewildering range of produce in the supermarket, vast amounts of information may offer patients a superficial illusion of perfect control and contentment, but in reality it signifies the commodification of care, and the further loss of community.

3 The wrong trousers

Admittedly, I did not look like a doctor. For one thing, I had just spent ten days on the Nile in a felucca with eight fellow travellers. (Feluccas are primitive sailing boats that look highly romantic in travel brochures but lose much of their allure on closer acquaintance). For another, when we reached Luxor, I had been struck by one of those acute delusional shopping disorders that so often afflict tourists, and purchased a pair of baggy cotton trousers with broad black and yellow stripes. I wore these for the rest of the journey south, so that by the time we boarded the overnight train from Aswan to Cairo I looked more like a dishevelled and overgrown bumble bee than a doctor.

'Is there a doctor on the train?' The message came over the public address system in Arabic, then French and then English. Aswan was a couple of hours behind us. I felt a strong a desire to deny my profession, but in the past two weeks I had already attended most of my fellow holidaymakers for the usual unpleasant ailments that go with so-called 'adventure travel', and they all knew what I did for a living. Wistfully, I recalled a consultant neurologist at my medical school who taught us exactly how to walk past a traffic accident on the other side of the street, but it was clear that on this occasion I could not put the teaching into practice.

Lurching along the corridor towards the back of the train, I found an edgy Egyptian guide attached to a party of French tourists who, judging by their dress and demeanour, had spent considerably more on their trip than we had on ours. They raised eyebrows at my ridiculous appearance, but allowed me to enter the compartment where I met the patient, a ten-year-old boy. He was accompanied by a male guardian who could have been an uncle or perhaps a private tutor. Both guardian and boy were pale and sweaty. In the guardian's case it was no doubt from anxiety. The boy, however, had a thin racing pulse and a rigid abdomen.

I explained that the child had peritonitis and needed urgent surgery. This provoked a frightening response. The Egyptian guide lost the few vestiges of restraint that had held her panic in check, and began to shout at me. I persisted, saying that the train would need to make an unscheduled halt at Luxor to let him and his guardian go to the hospital there. At this news the guardian practically passed out, while the guide dismissed my advice completely, saying that the hospitals were bad in Luxor and the child would be much safer waiting until we reached Cairo in about eighteen hours. I said as calmly as I could that he might die within eighteen hours, and that it was beyond belief that a town the size of

Luxor would not have a surgeon who could remove an appendix competently. Various members of the French party then came in to ask for proof that I really was a doctor. Close to losing my own temper, I managed to say witheringly: 'Je suis desolé, mais je ne porte pas mes diplômes en vacances'.

With bad grace, two of the French tourists finally agreed that they would discuss the matter with the guard, and then dismissed me. I returned to my own carriage. I had barely finished narrating the story to my own tour party and our Dutch guide, when another announcement came over the public address system. This time it was only in French, inquiring if there was a French doctor on the train. The stress was emphatically on the word 'français'.

I leapt up in disgust. This time, fortunately, our guide offered to come with me. He had displayed his equanimity already on the trip in various ways, and I knew that he spoke better French than me, as well as some Arabic. When we reached the boy's compartment we found, not surprisingly, that no French doctors had appeared, but a French nurse from another tour party had identified herself. She was, mercifully, an operating theatre nurse who must have seen hundreds of cases of peritonitis. Her elegance and fragrance also appeared to give her more professional authority than I could muster.

Through a series of negotiations that would not have disgraced Castlereagh or Talleyrand, it was agreed that I would re-examine the boy under the appraising eyes of the French nurse. I did so, and with a regal nod she indicated to her compatriots that, beneath my carnival outfit and uncouth appearance, I did indeed seem to be a doctor, and that the signs I had elicited were grave. At this point my guide urged me to return to my own companions. 'You have done your job as a doctor', he said impressively, 'and I will now do mine as your tour leader'. I supplied my name and surgery address to two of the more imperious Frenchmen at their request, unclear whether they wanted it for insurance purposes or with the intention of suing me if I turned out to have caused them any inconvenience. Then I left.

For about six months I heard nothing, but eventually received a letter from the boy's parents in France, offering their thanks. Their son had had an emergency appendicectomy in Luxor, and had been transferred to Cairo for postoperative care, where they had joined him. His recovery had been slow and complicated, but he was now quite well.

Later that year, I pottered around the garden in my bumble-bee trousers a couple of times, but then I put them in the fancy dress box in the loft, together with the loin cloth and spear from Kenya, the fez and pointed slippers from Marrakesh, and the Nigerian tribal outfit. I have never worn them since.

4 Darwin's dangerous idea

Most educated people nowadays know that we share over 98% of our DNA with chimpanzees. It does not disconcert us. The Victorians may have reacted with outrage to the proposition that we share our ancestors with the great apes, but we now live comfortably with the knowledge of our cousinhood.

We also share 50% of our DNA with bananas. This is a little harder to come to terms with. We cannot know how the bananas feel about it, but many humans may experience a *frisson* on learning this fact. The *frisson* may only be a faint echo of the existential horror that Darwin's contemporaries had to deal with. All the same, it gives us some sense of the blow that he delivered to their self-esteem.

Modern doctors have a somewhat peculiar relationship with Darwinism and evolutionary biology. The problem is not one of disbelief. Only a small minority of doctors still have anti-Darwinian views about the origin of species or the descent of man. No doubt they continue to defend these in the same way that the Inquisition challenged Galileo: by arguing that God wants to test our faith by scattering plausible illusions around the universe. However, most of us find little appeal or logic in the idea of a celestial Paul Daniels, or a transcendent Tommy Cooper.

The problem for doctors is perhaps more one of inattention. Evolutionary biology is like a background hum. It is always there but we never quite stop in order to hear it. We busy ourselves every day with its myriad manifestations – anatomy, physiology, molecular genetics or whatever – without noticing their implications. We may believe that we are thinking about the grander picture, but probably we are not.

Our attitudes to bacteria are a good example. As doctors we respect bacteria, both as adversaries and as commensals. We acknowledge that we cannot live without them, and that sometimes we cannot live with them either. Yet we systematically suppress the memory that they are something else to us as well. For a start, they spent several thousand million years manufacturing the atmosphere that made all later life forms possible. Then, they became the common ancestors for ourselves, chimpanzees, bananas and everything that grows and crawls on our planet. The microbiology reports that sit on our desk each morning are in fact the latest gossip about our distant grandparents, and tell us whether we and they are hitting it off. From the bacteria's perspective we are probably fulfilling our allotted role in the family pretty well, since we each carry around more of their cells than we do of our own.

We seem to have a similarly selective understanding of biochemistry too. At medical school we all learn the Krebs cycle. Later, it becomes a familiar litany or falls a victim to embarrassing amnesia. Either way, we scarcely pause to reflect that it too is only part of a much wider interactive picture: it has its inescapable counterpart in plant photosynthesis. Neither our cycle of phosphorylation nor theirs of photo-phosphorylation could survive without the other. As animals, we nourish ourselves on the waste gases of vegetables – bananas included – and they do on ours.

Why do we not hold these things in mind more often? Partly, it may be because of their enormity. For example, we can only make sense of the evolutionary time scale by likening it to a human life – with the earth as a 46-year-old person, and human civilization as the last two hours. In the same way, we can only concentrate on the effects of genetic mutations by turning our gaze away from the distant supernovae that, millions of years before, spat out the particles that caused those mutations.

The enormity is an intellectual one but it is an emotional one too. Psychoanalysts talk of the 'nameless dread' that every infant has to learn to contain in order to develop a coherent sense of self. It is a dread of fragmentation, of annihilation, of not-being. If we ever re-encounter this dread as adults (and most of us probably do at times) it may be when we try to assimilate the unassimilable. This must surely include any attempt to apprehend our position as a species in time and in space.

Darwin's readers had difficulty in accepting his evidence because it was inconsistent with their understanding of the past. Our own true difficulty with evolutionary biology may have more to do with the challenge it poses to our expectations about the future. So far as we know, we are the only species ever to have had foreknowledge of our own inevitable extinction, collectively as well as individually. We now know that we are not equipped to survive even the planetary glaciations that occur with breakneck frequency in evolutionary terms – let alone the cosmic collisions that have regularly wiped out 70% or more of all earthly creatures.

I sometimes find it puzzling that we do not insist on medical school applicants having biology even at GCSE, let alone at A level. Yet perhaps it is not so surprising. In spite of our apparently relaxed view of Darwin, we may not want to examine the implications of his discoveries, any more than the disgusted bishops and furious pamphleteers of his time. He posed theological challenges that still remain to be addressed. Thinking about them too much may take our minds off the job.

5 Personal services

At the end of our street there is a dry cleaning shop with the delightful name of *Etiquette*. The Turkish lady who runs it has been there for about 20 years, roughly the same length of time that I have lived in my house. In the past I had little to do with her, because I used a dry cleaner near my surgery, but last year I decided to start taking my clothes to Etiquette instead.

In the months I have been going there, the Turkish lady and I have developed a routine of repartee. She knows that I am a doctor (from the name on my cheques), and always asks if I am busy at work today. I make a great play of saying no, I am never busy. In fact, I tell her, I avoid work at all costs: perhaps I will do a locum surgery some time next week if I feel in the mood. Anyway, I explain, I spend most of the time telling other doctors what to do. It is less stressful than seeing patients, and earns me more money. The Turkish lady laughs, knowing that I am telling some kind of truth, but not the whole truth. If she asks me what kind of doctor I really am, I tell her that I am a pretty awful one, and I would certainly not recommend myself to any patients. But she asks me from time to time for advice about a medical problem in her family, and suddenly we both become serious for a while.

Very often, there is another lady in the shop, an English woman who appears to be a regular customer-cum-friend. Usually she seems ensconced there, sometimes with her own chair and a cup of coffee. She joins in our repartee as well, perhaps with an anecdote about some terrible doctor ('Most doctors are terrible', I am always happy to affirm.) I complain that the lady behind the counter never offers *me* a chair or a cup of coffee. The two of them cheerfully gang up on me and the talk then turns to women and friendship, versus men and business. All this time, other customers come and go, and most of them also seem to enjoy participating in the banter, like a game of verbal 'consequences', played by the whole community.

It has recently dawned on me that I always come out of Etiquette feeling happy. On mornings when I drop my clothes in on the way to work – for I do occasionally undertake work – it helps to set me up for the day. On late afternoons, when I collect them on the final stretch home, I feel a little revived. The dry cleaning shop is a place where I shed responsibility for a few minutes, and take on a personality of choice. It offers, I suppose, a form of therapy.

The dry cleaning lady, it has to be said, does not look like a therapist, but then few good therapists do. Yet I would not be at all surprised if she knows exactly what she is doing. Possibly she would be able to name the attributes that make her such a good therapist: curiosity, challenge, humour, a good memory, continuity of care – and of course etiquette. I wonder also if she makes the connection between her role as therapist and the care she gives to her clients' clothes. We take our soiled and crumpled clothing to her and she turns them back into spotless, comfortable and nicely pressed garments that we can be proud to wear. Sartorially, she is offering us a form of transformation, a symbolic washing away of our grimy everyday failings, a resurrection of hope, and new beginnings. And while she does so, maybe she is offering us the same thing conversationally as well.

We have quite a lot to learn from dry cleaners, and booksellers, and taxi drivers, and newsagents, and the hundreds of other people to whom we chatter away unthinkingly every day, under the mistaken impression that we are just passing the time and they are merely being polite. A hairdresser I spoke to the other day explained to me patiently the reasons why people trusted him more than they ever could their GPs: he is reliably available to them every time they book, he touches them physically on every occasion they see him, he is sensitive to their exact wishes, and he takes all the time they need. 'The thing is', he concluded, without any hint of irony or condescension, 'unlike your job, ours depends entirely on understanding psychology'. I suspect the dry cleaner at the end of the road might say much the same.

6 How not to be a doctor

'How can I help you?' I asked. It isn't the way I always open consultations but I was making a teaching video, so I thought I would be conventional for a change. As it turned out, it was a fortunate move. 'I'm not sure if you really *can* help me', the patient answered. 'I've seen lots of specialists, and none of them have managed to help me so far. You see, I keep having these funny turns ...' Two weeks later, when showing the video to a group of senior house officers, I stopped the recording at this point and asked them to write down the woman's presenting complaint. All ten of them wrote down 'funny turns.' They were wrong, of course. The woman's presenting problem was that she wasn't sure if I could really help her. The funny turns were at this point a lesser problem.

There were more shocks in store for the group. I spent almost the entire consultation asking the woman about her experience of other doctors, and what they had got wrong. I listened as dispassionately as I could, without dismissing her catalogue of disappointment or offering any hint that I might do any better myself. In the end I asked her what she thought the doctors ought to have done instead. She told me: a referral for homoeopathy or acupuncture. I asked her which of these she would prefer. She chose the homoeopathy referral, and I said I would arrange this. As she left, I thought she was going to cry with relief.

After I had finished showing the video, one junior doctor erupted. How could I have been so incompetent – not to take a full history, or indeed any history at all? How could I be so irresponsible, by assuming that the other doctors had not done their job properly? How could I be certain that her funny turns did not presage some terrible, terminal disease? If I thought the problem was psychosomatic, why didn't I take a decent psychiatric history instead? And how could I possibly direct her, without a clear diagnosis, towards a form of treatment that I probably didn't believe in, and which lacked a thorough evidence base?

A number of other doctors in the group came to my defence. Some had realized that I might have looked at the notes in advance, and that I might be willing to trust local colleagues not to make gross errors of judgement. Others had heard the patient mention that she had gone through the mill of extensive and futile investigations several times over. One or two had noticed how the patient gave indications of an aversion to anything remotely suggesting psychological inquiry. A particularly thoughtful doctor pointed out that no intervention was without its risks; at this stage it would probably cause the patient more risk if I started all over again, instead of just doing what she wanted. Yet their sceptical colleague remained unconvinced. How could I have behaved so ... so ... well, so unlike a doctor? I took the question as a compliment.

Of all professions, doctors are almost invariably the most proficient at not listening. Indeed, a friend of mine sometimes describes my educational work in consultation skills as 'remedial therapy for selective brain damage'. It is a cruel characterization, but I do not entirely object to it. I am struck again and again by how much medical listening – even the kind that sometimes passes for being 'patient-centred' – falls desperately short of anything that one might expect from an attentive, untrained friend. Many doctors seem to tune out totally from any words or phrases that do not fit the medical construction of the world. In addition, most appear to be extraordinarily timid about going where the patient wants to lead, for fear that this will break some rule, or upset any other doctor who might hear about it.

When it comes to unexplained symptoms, I often observe doctors fall back on an impoverished list of questions such as 'are you under any stress?' rather than displaying any true curiosity about the story itself. There are two other common consultation ploys that bring me out in an allergic reaction. One is the question 'How did you *feel* about that?'. It is generally asked as the doctor asking leans forward in a theatrical pose of solicitousness, but with eyes glazed over in weary automatism. The question seems to go with a belief that it will elicit some definitional nugget of truth, accompanied by a sublime catharsis on the part of the patient. It arises, I guess, from some ghastly misreading of Freud's more minor followers, but ninety-nine times out of a hundred, it is emotionally bogus. The other manoeuvre that I find equally offensive is the phrase 'It *sounds* as if ...' (as in 'it sounds as if you're very upset ...'). Believe me, if it's so obvious that even a doctor has noticed, it usually isn't worth saying.

Lois Shawver, a Californian therapist and teacher whom I much respect, has come up with a wonderful distinction between 'listening in order to speak' and 'speaking in order to listen.' In the former, you merely scan the words that patients are saying, looking for opportunities to dive in and tell them what is 'really' going on. In the latter, you do the opposite: speaking only in order to give them more opportunities to explain their own view of the world. In a post-modern age where the authority of professional knowledge is gradually waning away, Shawver argues that we will have to learn how to speak less and listen more.

In the same vein, the late Harry Goolishian, one of the founders of narrative approaches to psychiatry, offered the advice: 'Don't listen to what patients mean, listen to what they say!' Quite simple really, except that we probably still fail to do this, most of the time.

7 Modern medicine

6.30 am. Woken by the alarm clock before the morning chorus. The roads are pretty clear on my way in, so for a change I manage to find a place in the main hospital car park, opposite the one reserved for the director of finance.

7.45 am. A working breakfast with the chief executive and medical director. Apparently they want me to re-write the section about my unit in the Trust's annual report. Bob, the CEO, comments that it is 'too factual'. Sarah – once my registrar, now the MD – suggests that we should cut out a lot of the text and replace it with nice photos: she knows a good agency that provides these. I argue the toss for a while, but they manage to convince me that good PR is an absolute necessity for hospitals these days. I couldn't help noticing how well Bob and Sarah are getting on. I can remember how she used to call me 'sir', but now she is the only one apart from my mother who calls me Charlie instead of Charles.

8.30 am. I attend the first shift in this year's CPR training. Evidently the old mantra of 'ABC' – airways, breathing and circulation – has gone the way of the dinosaurs. The nurse running the session tells us a much longer and more helpful mnemonic, which I forget for the moment, but I have written it down in my Filofax. (Apparently I am the last doctor in the Trust who still has a Filofax instead of one of those electronic things with a large toothpick. I shall ask my children to get me one for Christmas, and no doubt their own children can teach me how to use it.) Bob is at the training session too and makes an ass of himself by saying that he would maintain cardiac massage in preference to applying pressure to an arterial wound in someone who is haemorrhaging to death. Odd, when you consider he used to be an anaesthetist.

10.00 am. Just in time for a meeting of the ethnicity and diversity sub-committee, which I now chair (Sarah can be very persuasive when she puts her mind to it. When we did my job plan she said something about it being a bit lightweight: 'just seeing lots of patients and dabbling in research, but not much else'). There is a big agenda. We commission some very useful statistical reviews covering everything from consultants' discretionary points to ethnic monitoring of our car park staff – who were accidentally left off last month's survey. This business of ethnic monitoring is another area where I used to be less than politically correct, but I got an ear-bashing over this from Bob's new young wife at a dinner party a while ago, and I am now thoroughly on message about it.

11.30 am. I get to the next meeting by the skin of my teeth. It is a mandatory fire and safety training that I signed up for several weeks ago. I feel rather ashamed of myself because I seem to have forgotten the difference between the three different types of fire extinguisher. The fire officer who does the presentation is an absolute wizard with PowerPoint, and I am a bit surprised when he mentions that he no longer works on the front line as a fireman. He looks quite a fit young man.

1.00 pm. Lunch. I always used to miss this and eat on the hoof, but the inspectors from the Health Commission visited us earlier in the year and noticed 'a culture of comfort grazing rather than a model of healthy eating', so nowadays I am careful to be seen in the canteen. I hold a conversation in the queue with two of our honoraries who tell me that they are introducing a system of 'educational governance' for everyone involved with the training grades. I am of course familiar with clinical governance and research governance, but I must confess I have been training my juniors on the old principle of 'sitting by Nellie'. I shall try to pull my socks up and go to a few meetings about this. Sadly my lunch break means that I don't get time to record the morning's activities for my appraisal folder. I also feel rather embarrassed afterwards to discover that I missed a lunchtime meeting on detecting poor performance in colleagues.

1.30 pm. Most of the afternoon is taken up with the serious business of building up our patient liaison service. I am now the consultant rep on this (Sarah's influence again – what is it about that woman?) We have to interview a number of candidates from the local community to join us. It is a formidable task. Fortunately our head of human resources has already done a 'comprehensive mapping exercise of local stakeholders', and she brings along a very thorough set of government guidelines about making such appointments. We take an hour just to familiarize ourselves with these, but in the end we manage to appoint some good people. Evidently there is a very robust appeals procedure for anyone who feels unfairly rejected.

4.30 pm. All our non-medical staff are in the process of having their contracts revised: something to do with modernization and Europe, I think, although I am not entirely clear about this. Consultant medical staff are exempt, but I was touched when the union shop steward asked if I would give some input. (I was rather touched to discover that there still *was* a shop steward.) Unfortunately at the meeting itself I find that I don't really have much to contribute. My suggestion that 'Operating Theatre Assistant' remains a better term than 'Parasurgical Resource Officer Grade One' does not win favour. Apparently Bob is very keen on 'rebranding', Sarah even more so.

5.30 pm. There is a note on my desk when I return to my office. One of my more vulnerable patients has apparently phoned up in a state and left a message with my secretary. 'He says he is pretty desperate,' she has written, 'and would be terribly grateful if you could phone as soon as possible.' I pick up the receiver, but then suddenly remember the tremendous telling-off we had all had from Sarah (and Bob) about not sticking to the Working Time Directive. Apparently our next rating in the league table may hinge on this. Reluctantly, I replace the receiver. I shall have to make the call tomorrow – if my other commitments permit.

8 Plus ça change...

Og and Nyp sat by the fire outside the cave. Og, the older of the two medicine men, chewed hungrily at a metatarsal taken from the mammoth that the clan had hunted down the previous day. Nyp sat quietly, staring into the dying embers of the fire.

'Medicine?' Og said with scorn in his voice. 'It isn't medicine as I remember it. In the old days, if a man was possessed by an evil spirit, you knew what a medicine man had to do. You consulted with the ancestors in your dreams. Then you did what they told you. You took a good flint arrowhead and a big stone, and you walloped a damn good hole into the man's skull. Next morning, he got up feeling right as rain, and the evil spirit had gone away.'

'And what happens nowadays?' Og spat a piece of mammoth gristle contemptuously into the ashes. 'You have to go to all the elders of the clan, and ask their permission. They talk and they talk. They even ask the women what they think, for goodness' sake. Then one elder tells you that everyone these days is using bigger arrowheads and smaller stones. Another says the hole mustn't be wider than a baby's little finger. Some busybody – who wouldn't know an evil spirit if it smacked him in the face – says he's worried what the family will do if the sick person dies. Then everyone starts to prattle about the family's right to take retribution on you. Retribution! On a medicine man! Have you ever heard of anything so preposterous?'

Og reached into the pile of mammoth bones, helped himself to a clavicle, grasped it in both hands, and started to gnaw at it greedily. Nyp kept silent. He had heard Og talk like this before. He had great respect for Og and for all the medicine men of that generation. Before them, medicine had been truly Neanderthal. Now, thanks to men like Og, all of that had changed. It was impossible to imagine that mashed beetle poultices and infusions of ground sabre tooth had been totally unknown when Og had himself been a young man. How could one possibly have practised medicine without them? And when disease had decimated the clan, Nyp had seen Og in person sacrifice captives to the ancestors, with an elegance that took your breath away. But the world was changing, and men like Og could never halt progress.

'I tell you one of the worst things,' Og carried on. 'In the old days, if a man was possessed and his local medicine man couldn't expel the spirit with simple remedies, you used to go to the victim's cave yourself. You thought nothing of it. When did you last hear of anyone doing that? They're all too bloody self-important these days. No one does cave visits any more.'

'You could tell a lot from a cave, you know. You could see at once if the gods wanted someone to live or die. You looked at the paintings on the walls, for instance. They showed you a hell of a lot, those paintings. If all you saw was a charcoal sketch, with a few pathetic skinny rabbits, you didn't much fancy the patient's chances against an evil spirit. On the other hand, if you saw a bison hunt, drawn to last a few years maybe, you knew you were in business.'

Nyp had heard the arguments before but he wasn't convinced. He had seen these caves. Some were utterly disgusting, really unspeakable. They certainly weren't the kind of places you could sit down and grind together a decent mixture of wolf dung, fresh slugs and boar sperm, or any of the other cleansing potions that people liked to swallow these days.

Og tore one last morsel off the clavicle and then hesitated between a rib and a tibia. He chose the tibia. He ate a few mouthfuls and then spoke again. 'Actually, there's something even worse than cave visits dying out. It's this new-fangled obsession with growing things. Our forefathers found plants for medicines just like they found their food. They picked things up from where the gods had left them. Nowadays you young people think you can steal the seeds and put them in the ground yourself. Then you just sit on your backsides and watch the plants come up. Tell me, do you honestly call that natural?'

'What next, I ask you?' he continued. 'Soon you'll be capturing rams and forcing them to copulate with their ewes and make lambs to order, because you can't be bothered to lift a spear to catch your dinner. What kind of life would *that* be?'

Nyp sighed. The old man was getting carried away now, and just talking nonsense. By now, Og had finished his tibia and he was stretching his arm out again towards the pile of bones. Nyp had had enough. 'Old man,' he said, 'you eat too much mammoth meat. It isn't good for your health.'

9 Anna O and the 'talking cure'

'At the time of her falling ill (in 1880) Fräulein Anna O was twenty-one years old'. Thus begins one of the most famous of all case histories.[1] Its author was Dr Josef Breuer. A kind, cultivated and generous man, Breuer was one of the most distinguished physicians of his time, and he counted the great surgeon Theodor Billroth among his patients. He was also an eminent neurophysiologist and discovered the action of the vagus nerve on respiration, as well as the function of the semicircular canals. For some years he engaged a young man named Sigmund Freud to work in his laboratory at the university of Vienna, and it was Freud who eventually managed to persuade him to publish the details of Anna's illness and treatment.

Anna, according to Breuer, 'had hitherto been consistently healthy and had shown no signs of neurosis during her period of growth. She was markedly intelligent, with an astonishingly quick grasp of things and penetrating intuition. She had great poetic gifts, which were under the control of a sharp and critical common sense.' In spite of these attributes, Breuer reported, Anna fell prey, during her father's final illness and in the months after his death, to the most appalling symptoms of hysterical paralysis and anaesthesia in three out of her four limbs, together with a succession of other distressing psychiatric symptoms. At different times these included weakness, inability to turn her head, diplopia, a nervous cough, loss of appetite, hallucinations, agitation, mood swings, abusive and destructive behaviour, amnesia, somnolence, tunnel vision and partial aphasia ('She no longer conjugated verbs', Breuer recorded, 'and eventually she used only infinitives, for the most part incorrectly formed from weak past participles'). Among her symptoms, she was at one time unable to speak in her native German, but could still read both French and Italian, translating them aloud into English as she did so. During part of her illness, she was unable to recognize or accept food from anyone except her physician, who spent somewhere in the region of a thousand hours with her between April 1881 and June 1882. She was able to satisfy herself of his identity only by holding his hands.

As described by Dr Breuer, his treatment of Anna gradually developed through three stages, as he responded to Anna's own apparent wishes. In the first stage, he recognized that she could relieve her distress by making up and telling fairy tales, 'always sad and some of them very charming' – and he encouraged her to do so. She herself called this activity 'chimney sweeping' or her 'talking cure' (the origin of this famous term for all later forms of psychotherapy and counselling). In the second stage, Breuer was able to hypnotize Anna every morning, sometimes by holding up an orange, in order to help her to remember some of the painful emotions she had gone through when her father was dying. Each evening Breuer would return and Anna would recount, with vivid emotion, the exact events from precisely one year previously. In the final stage, Anna began to add to these accounts a description of the various occurrences that had evidently triggered each of her hysterical symptoms during the previous year. As she did so, the relevant symptom itself would disappear. For example, on recalling her disgust at seeing a dog drink from a lady companion's glass of water a year before, she was suddenly able to drink once more, having for some time been able to quench her thirst only by eating fruit such as melons.

Breuer's history of Anna O has given rise to a tremendous amount of debate. There seems to be much uncertainty about the true extent of Anna's clinical improvement following the treatment. We know that Anna was admitted to a sanatorium shortly after her apparent 'cure', still in a very disturbed state – although in later life she became a distinguished social worker and a noted campaigner for women's rights (under her real name of Bertha Pappenheim). Freud himself was the first to criticize Breuer for his naïveté, in particular for ignoring Anna's fairly obvious sexual feelings towards her physician. Breuer himself, if not actually infatuated with Anna, certainly seems to have been drawn into a kind of 'folie à deux', accepting her behaviour and her self-prescribed cures at face value, and discounting the effect of his own intense interest on her performance. It has also been suggested that Anna's theatrics drew heavily on the contemporary craze in Vienna for stage hypnotism.[2] For many modern readers, it may be quite hard to avoid the impression of an annoying young woman running rings around a rather suggestible doctor.

However, it may be worth reflecting on this reaction a little, and applying some historical sensitivity to what we read. If Anna's hysteria appears to us now as a form of outrageous fabrication, it may be for the simple reason that she had lost the capacity either to know the truth or to tell it. In addition, within her own cultural world such 'mad' behaviour was one of the few permissible forms of protest open to young women who felt stultified by their family and social circumstances. (There was opposition, for example, to girls receiving secondary education. Billroth himself was against it, on the grounds that it might lead to demands for women to enter the university.) Seen from this kind of perspective, her girlish determination to engage her physician with a bizarre drama of symptoms and remedies does indeed represent a shocking state of mind, and a desperate plea for relief. When Breuer approached Anna's bedside with an apparently obsessive interest in the tiniest details of her behaviour, he was displaying the most objective and enlightened stance available to a medical man of his time, not to mention a great deal of patience and devotion. What Breuer did was in fact utterly original in relation to any form of mental distress: he listened not only in order to establish a diagnosis, but also to effect a treatment. Freud, for all his reservations about the case, realised how radical this was, and drew on it for the basis of his own talking cure. If, with hindsight, we regard

Breuer's view of these events (and even Freud's) as somewhat selective and self-promoting, this may be no more the case than with many other scientific advances.

We live now in a world that is united, if at all, by the idea that talking does indeed cure. Whether as doctors or therapists, our daily experience is that letting people talk does make a difference. Few if any psychotherapists these days believe, like Breuer, that prompting patients to recall trivial events from the recent past will alleviate psychosomatic symptoms. Most believe that talking works because it provides people with a means of creating a coherent narrative from disconnected symptoms, events, memories and thoughts in the context of a relationship with someone compassionate and attentive. Whether this relationship lasts for a single medical consultation, or a long course of therapy, it may help to correct some of the hurt done by less well-attuned relationships, or by significant losses and setbacks, and to make sense of them. What is particularly interesting is that a growing amount of collaborative research, done by neuroscientists and psychiatrists working together, suggests that such processes may bring about demonstrable changes at a neurological level.[3] If this is true, we may have come full circle. It would no doubt have delighted Dr Josef Breuer, physician and physiologist, who held Bertha Pappenheim's hands, listened to her fairy stories and took them seriously.

1. Breuer J. Fräulein Anna O. In: Freud S. *The Standard Edition of the Complete Psychological Works of Sigmund Freud*, Vol II (ed. Strachey J). London, Hogarth Press, 1955.
2. Borch-Jacobsen M. *Remembering Anna O: A century of mystification.* London, Routledge, 1996.
3. Kaplan-Solms K, Solms M. *Clinical Studies in Neuro-Psychoanalysis.* London, Karnac, 2000.

10 Breaking the news

We all commiserated as our colleague told us about her awful consultation the previous day. She had had to tell a man in his fifties that his ultrasound scan had shown a mass in the head of his pancreas, almost certainly a carcinoma. The man clearly hadn't been expecting bad news, and had turned up at the surgery on his own, with a rather jaunty manner. To make matters worse, she had never met the man previously – she was covering for someone else that day. We squirmed and offered our sympathy as she described the encounter unfolding from moment to moment. She was honest enough to admit that she hadn't actually liked the man, who had been a bit smelly. At the end of the consultation she had wanted to hug him, or at the very least to touch him on the arm, but found herself unable to. We were all experienced educators as well as clinicians, and we tried to cover every angle in our discussion: the painfully inappropriate circumstances in which we often have to break bad news; the way in which negative impressions can disable our compassion; and how we aspire to the impossible task of spelling out a death sentence nicely, and feel like failures when it never quite happens that way.

Yet afterwards I pondered on her story and I couldn't get another, heretical thought out of my mind: *why did the doctor have to tell the truth?* There must have been a dozen ways in which she might have delayed or underplayed telling the man the full scan result, at least until a relative could be present – or until the patient's usual doctor was available. It took little imagination to think of various forms of subterfuge that she might have used: 'the result isn't back yet ...', 'it's back but it's not entirely clear ...', 'I'm a bit puzzled about its significance and I need to discuss it with a colleague ...' If such prevarications had raised the patient's anxiety, would that have been so terrible, especially by comparison with what actually did happen? I recalled that a generation ago, few doctors would ever have dreamed of telling this man the truth in this way. And surely no group of experienced doctors at that time would have failed to mention, or even to think, that it might have been done differently.

Autres temps, autres moeurs. But culture makes a difference too. A week later, I was teaching a group of interpreters and linkworkers, mainly from eastern Europe. The same theme arose again. One of them described, with horror, how a friend of hers had been to see a doctor in London who had told him – 'by himself, on the spot, there and then' – that he had a lymphoma. Back home, she said, no-one would ever give someone such information without first checking with the family whether the patient had the resilience to absorb it, or to cope with it. When she said this, her peer group murmured their agreement, and by implication expressed their disapproval of the brutal and uncompromising frankness of British doctors.

As it happens, her views find support in cross-cultural research about death and dying. In many parts of the world, and among many cultures, people still take a far more circumspect approach to the disclosure of a terminal illness than we generally now do in the West. According to medical anthropologists and family researchers, this may have nothing to do with paternalism or with a fear of being honest. Instead, it may arise from a belief in the crucial importance of sustaining hope as a life force, together with a radically different understanding of the duties of the individual towards the family and vice versa.

'In cultures where the family is the unit of identity and responsibility,' writes Lucy Candib from the University of Massachusetts, 'interdependence is the higher value, not individualism ... The patient knows that family is protecting her and that this is what families should do ... Non-disclosure is not a matter of lying. Ambiguity may be seen as the most suitable strategy to allow the patient to maintain tranquillity'.[1] Candib cautions us, however, against making simplistic assumptions that everyone from within a certain culture will share the same preference for or against knowing the truth. She advises physicians to 'offer the option of truth' when breaking bad news, regardless of where the patient comes from. She suggests using questions such as these: 'Will you want to be making the decisions about your care with the doctors, or do you want your family to be making those decisions?' and 'When we understand what is causing your illness, will you want us to tell you about it, or to talk with your family about it?'

This kind of sensitivity to cultural and individual norms is gaining increasing support among medical ethicists. Following several decades of so-called 'principlist' ethics (based on the four well-known principles of autonomy, non-maleficence, beneficence and justice), an increasing number of theorists now seem to be moving towards a more flexible and relativist approach known as 'narrative ethics'. One of the central tenets of this approach is that every situation is unique and unrepeatable, and cannot be fully captured by appealing to universal principles.[2] Any decision or action is therefore justified in terms of its fit with the individual life story of the patient, and needs to be sought through conversation rather than based on prior notions. Narrative ethics also 'encourages multiple voices to be heard and multiple stories to be brought forth by all those whose lives will be involved in the resolution of a case. Patient, physician, family, health professional, friend and social worker, for example, may all share their stories in a dialogical chorus that can offer the best chance of respecting all the persons involved in a case'.[3]

Seen in this light, our colleague's assumption that there was only one right action when faced with the jaunty man with pancreatic cancer might be seen as an example of die-hard principlism, with an excessive bias towards the notion of autonomy. But then again, to be entirely fair to her, where can most of us find a 'dialogical chorus' to help us with our ethical dilemmas, on an average working day in the National Health Service?

1. Candib L. Truth telling and advance planning at the end of life: problems with autonomy in a multi-cultural world. *Fam Syst Health* 2002; **20**:213–28.
2. McCarthy J. Principlism or narrative ethics: must we choose between them? *J Med Ethics: Medical Humanities* 2003; **29**:65–71.
3. Hudson Jones A. Narrative in medical ethics. In: Greenhalgh T, Hurwitz B, eds. *Narrative Based Medicine: Dialogue and discourse in clinical practice.* London, BMJ Books, 1998.

11 Cultural nepotism

Do you know who first discovered the systemic circulation of the blood? Of course you do. He was an Englishman called William Harvey. But can you name the person who, three centuries earlier, first described the pulmonary circulation? Almost certainly not. He was a Syrian Arab physician by the name of Ibn al-Nafis. The writings of al-Nafis were probably known to Michael Servetus, whose own understanding of the pulmonary vessels paved the way for Harvey's theory.

If this example of Eurocentrism in our knowledge of history was a fairly isolated one, it would be no great matter. The problem, however, is that our general ignorance in Western countries of Islamic history is so comprehensive and so massive that it has led us into a world view that it may be no exaggeration to describe as delusional.

For a thousand years, from the victories of the caliph Omar in the seventh century to the retreat of the Ottomans from Vienna in the seventeenth, civilization from the Atlantic to beyond the Indian Ocean was predominantly Islamic. Our Dark Ages and Middle Ages were the obverse of what was a glorious millennium in the Muslim world. We often regard the Roman world as the yardstick for the size and duration of cultures, but it was a relatively modest presentiment of what the conquering Muslims later achieved, and it came and went in little more than four centuries. (Even this degree of longevity has yet to be achieved by the succession of brief European empires that have prevailed since the Ottomans retreated: those of Spain, Portugal, England, Holland, Sweden, France, Austria, Germany, Russia and the USA.)

In all the arts and sciences, and in mathematics and philosophy, the achievements of Islamic culture during its ten centuries of primacy surpassed anything that had been known previously in history. Islamic thinkers believed themselves – with justification – to be the successors of all the earlier civilisations that had arisen in the Middle East, going back to the dawn of recorded history. For them, Baghdad was in a direct line of succession from nearby Babylon and ancient Ur. Yet they were also the inheritors of Greek knowledge, and in time they became the chief source of such knowledge for the Western Renaissance.

It is hard to get a sense from the written word or the historical atlas of the richness of Islamic civilisation, but anyone who has visited one of its great centres will have come away with an impression of a certain grace and serenity that, for all their greatness, cannot be found even in Paris or in Venice. If you want to risk a seismic shock to your cultural prejudices, I would recommend the walk from the ethereal courtyards of the Alhambra in Granada, built by the Moorish kings of Spain, down the hill to the gloomy cathedral that Ferdinand and Isabella built to celebrate the 'reconquest', ghoulishly furnished with images of torture and death.

An experience like this makes it possible to comprehend classical Islam's estimation of itself, and of the West. By and large, Islam saw itself, until modern times, as the definitive climax of all previous civilisations. Europe, by contrast, was seen to be sunk in superstitious barbarism – an impression that was confirmed periodically by the murderous but generally incompetent incursions of crusader warlords. The same contrast seemed evident in the levels of religious tolerance displayed in the Islamic and Western worlds. Moorish Spain, for example, was a golden age of cross-cultural synergy. It produced the great Hebrew poet Solomon Ibn Gabirol and the even greater philosopher Maimonides – both of whom wrote with equal fluency in Arabic. Later, while Europe was locked into the vicious wars of the Reformation and Counter-Reformation, the Mughal emperor Akbar was sponsoring interfaith dialogues involving Jesuits and Hindus in his court at Fatehpur Sikri. The Ottoman empire was for many centuries a place of refuge for the victims of religious persecution in Europe.

In the words of the historian Bernard Lewis, non-Muslims within the Islamic world generally experienced 'the normal constraints and occasional hazards of minority status'. However, as Lewis also points out, there is nothing in Islamic history to compare with the Spanish Inquisition, the *auto da fe*, the wars of religion, 'not to speak of more recent crimes of commission and acquiescence'. Against such a historical background, he argues, it becomes possible to empathize with the perplexity and pain of many contemporary Muslims. There is perplexity at the speed and completeness with which Western military power, technology and secular governance eventually swept aside a millennium of Islamic primacy on the world stage. But more than this, there is pain at the Western capacity to denigrate the Islamic past or to deny it altogether, and at our capacity to see Western acts of violence as aberrant or merely reactive, while we regard that of the Muslim world as pathognomonic or definitional.[1]

There may be no time better than the present for Western medical historians to honour Ibn al-Nafis, who died around the age of eighty and bequeathed his house, his estate and his library to a hospital in Cairo. We should also mourn Michael Servetus, who was arrested in 1553 in Geneva for his theories of physiology, and charged with heresy and blasphemy. He refused to retract, and was burned alive the next day. I suspect that many Muslims, both now and then, would not learn of this violent, irrational and misplaced reaction with any great surprise.

1. Lewis B. *What went wrong? Western impact and middle-eastern response.* London, Weidenfeld and Nicholson, 2002.

12 Doing the rounds

One of the greatest figures in the history of British hospitals in the twentieth century was not a doctor, but a former steelworker from Glasgow who later became a social worker and then a film maker. His name was James Robertson.

Robertson started his researches into paediatric wards in Britain in 1948. At that time, sick children were routinely separated from their parents for long periods of time. Having parents in hospital was regarded as disruptive, and staff were upset to hear how children cried when mothers arrived or left. Visits were restricted and in some cases forbidden. Here, for example, is a list of the visiting times in some of London's main hospitals from around that time, published in a survey in the *Spectator*:

'Guys Hospital, Sundays 2–4pm; St Bartholomew's, Wednesdays 2–3.30pm; St Thomas's, first month no visits, but parents could see their children asleep 7–8 pm; Westminster, Wednesdays, 2–3pm; West London, no visiting; Charing Cross, Sundays, 2–3pm; London Hospital, under three years old, no visits but parents could see through partitions, over three years old, twice weekly.'

The story of Robertson's campaign to change this state of affairs sheds no glory on hospitals, doctors or the British establishment. His meticulous researches into the effects of separation on children – distrust, rejection, wetting, soiling, anxiety and rages – were dismissed as sensational. The film he made with his wife Joyce to demonstrate these effects was shown at the Royal Society of Medicine in 1952 to unanimous derision, and to accusations of rigging. BBC producers blocked his attempts to present it on television. When they finally relented in 1961 and allowed him to show some excerpts, Robertson defied their orders by turning to the live camera to explain that parents had a legal right to stay with their children regardless of any 'official' rules. His courage inspired a group of mothers to form the National Association for the Welfare of Children in Hospital, one of the most effective pressure groups ever to have arisen. As a result of their work, there are probably no paediatric wards in Britain nowadays with any restrictions at all on parental visiting.

I find Robertson's story inspiring but also outrageous. The list of hospital visiting times, in particular, is heartbreaking. It makes me go hot and cold with anger, misery and a retrospective sense of helplessness. The emotional effects of such institutionalized brutality are too painful to hold in the imagination. How on earth can it have happened? How can people have believed that it was a good thing? How could doctors and nurses have been so blind to the distress they were causing, and so uncritical of themselves?

The answer, of course, is that the rules were familiar, and familiarity breeds conformism. As Robertson found, protests against convention can invite ridicule, particularly from the medical profession. We also need to remind ourselves of innumerable other examples of social practices that were considered humane for considerable periods of time, but that now fill us with horror – including slavery, workhouses, and large mental asylums in remote rural locations.

Which brings us, somewhat uncomfortably, to the question of whether there are any current practices that doctors now accept with complacency, but ought to regard as similarly grotesque. My own nomination for such a practice would be the ward round.

Before you accuse me of descending from the sublime to the ridiculous, let me explain that I have been a hospital in-patient myself several times, so I know from experience what it feels like to lie horizontally, in ill-fitting hospital pyjamas, while a large group of well-dressed and vertical doctors (some of whom have never introduced themselves) stand half out of earshot, discussing your life expectancy in a mixture of whispers, circumlocutions and euphemisms. More distressingly, I have seen my normally dignified wife subjected to the same humiliation by groups of mainly male colleagues, while I was dismissed from her bedside. And when my parents were alive, I observed each of them reduced to a similar state of humiliation, bewilderment, and more or less utter disempowerment each time they were in hospital and were victims of this uncaring but unchallengeable ritual.

In all these situations, I have wondered how it could still be permissible for patients to pass through their entire admissions to hospital without ever having the basic human dignity of one-to-one meetings with their doctors, sitting in a private space such as a ward office or day room, properly clothed if possible, and with family members present if they wished. I also find it dispiriting that some consultants manage to complete their entire careers without ever engaging in a single medical encounter of this kind with an in-patient (except possibly in their private practices). I am puzzled as to why hospital teams cannot allocate one main doctor to each in-patient so that this can happen.

From the perspective of general practice, confidential encounters between a single doctor and a patient or family are the cornerstone of good medical and emotional care. There seems no reason, beyond professional convention and convenience, why this cannot happen in hospitals too. Even frail and elderly patients can in most cases be helped to dress properly and to come alone into an office – with the help of a wheelchair if necessary – so that they can disclose their fears and articulate their questions in relative dignity. For the few who cannot, it is perfectly possible for any doctor to draw up a chair to the bedside on each visit. The medical team can of course still meet, as some already do, to discuss the 'case' quite separately from arranging for one sole doctor to meet the actual person face to face.

I wonder if we will have to wait for a latter day James Robertson so that this happens, or whether our own profession could seize the initiative in bringing the time-honoured but demeaning practice of ward rounds to an end. Is it wildly unrealistic to think that medical professors might take the lead?

13 The descent of man

1. These are the generations of man. In the beginning was deoxyribonucleic acid which begat more deoxyribonucleic acid, like unto itself.
2. And Lo, there were rays from the heavens, and mutation came to pass. And the deoxyribonucleic acid begat unicellular organisms, which we call prokaryotes. And there was variation amongst them, and competition, so that some thrived; but others vanished from the earth, which we call natural selection.
3. And prokaryotes multiplied upon the face of the earth: the true bacteria and also the mitochondria and the chloroplasts; and the archaebacteria. And the mitochondria and chloroplasts knew the prokaryotes, and they cleaved to one another. And together they begat the eukaryotes, which were nucleated cells. But the prokaryotes are the inheritors of the earth to this day.
4. Now the eukaryotes multiplied greatly, and they begat sixty or more lineages of protozoans, red algae, flagellates, ciliates, diatoms, brown algae, giardia, slime moulds, slime nets, red seaweeds and other wonderful creatures; but also they begat the opisthokonts, which is the name of the begetter of the creature that begat the plants, and which also begat the microsporidia and the fungi, and the choanoflagellates, and the metazoa, which we call animals.
5. And the plants and animals and fungi are close kin, and together they have departed from the other lineages.
6. The animals also knew each other in their day. Over the generations they divided amongst themselves and begat sponges and placozoa, and also the eumetazoa who are the comb-jellies, as well as the cnidarians that we call jellyfish, sea anemones, corals and hydra. And the eumetazoa had tissues and organs. And they also begat the bilateria, which are the same on the left and on the right and have three layers of cells, and among these are many worms, and we too are the children of worms.
7. Now the bilateria begat two great nations of worms who were the protostomes. These were the lophotrochozoa, which begat the molluscs, earthworms, leeches and their many kindred; and the ecdysozoa, which begat the roundworms and also the arthropods or insects, who are in number like the stars in the heavens. Among them too are spiders and crabs and their many kindred.
8. But also the bilateria begat the deuterostomes, whose anus is created through gastrulation before its mouth. And the deuterostomes are also in the likeness

of worms. And we are of the deuterostomes, because when we are newly formed in our mothers' wombs, yea, our anuses are open even before our mouths.

9. After some time, the deuterostomes begat the echinoderms which are the sea urchins and starfish and many others too; also the hemichordates; and the chordates, whose back is stiffened by a rod and who have a dorsal nerve. The chordates begat the generations of the urochordates and the amphioxus and lancelet; but also the chordates begat the vertebrates who have a spine.

10. And among the vertebrates are all the fishes: the hagfish and ostracoderms, which have neither skulls nor jaws, and the lamprey, which has a skull but no jaws. And there are many other creatures among the vertebrates, but also the gnathastomata, which have both a skull and jaws, as we do, being of a kin with such fish.

11. Now the gnathastomata begat many more fishes: the rays and sharks were of this kind. And after the generations some begat sarcopterygii, or lobe-finned fishes. The lobe-finned fishes divided too: some begat coelacanths and other creatures of the deep, but also there were terrestrial vertebrates, which were a miracle to behold, as they had limbs with digits and they could walk on land, verily as we do.

12. Among the terrestrial vertebrates were many stegocephalians, who have lungs and can hear; and also tetrapods, who have no inner gills, and also five fingers and toes on each limb. And the tetrapods begat the amphibians and reptilomorphs. As for ourselves, we are the children of the reptilomorphs.

13. The reptilomorphs divided among themselves and some begat amniotes. And of the amniotes there were reptilia, among whom were many of the dinosaurs, who later begat the birds. And a great rock came from the heavens, and a dark cloud passed over the earth. This was not the first great rock from the heavens, neither was it the last. And the dinosaurs passed away from the face of the earth, even as we shall.

14. But also among the reptilia were lizards, crocodiles and turtles. Moreover there were also amniotes called synapsids, who begat many creatures that sprawled like reptiles but were not of their kind. The synapsids in their day also begat the therapsids, who were like mammals but their young did not suckle. Yet therapsids also begat the mammals, whose young did suckle, and of such are we.

15. Of the mammals some begat monotremes, but others begat marsupials and placental mammals. The placental mammals were the eutheria and some begat anteaters and pangolins, hares and squirrels, pigs, and also whales who are close kin of the hippopotami, and others of their kind. Also they begat hedgehogs and tigers, and the ungulates, which we call boars and dolphins, aardvarks and rhinoceri, elephants and manatees, and great numbers of other creatures.

16. And some others of the eutheria went their way and begat bats, colugos and tree shrews. And we are among these, being very like tree shrews in our form and spirit, even unto this day.

17. Now the tree shrews begat primates, and the primates begat the lemurs and bush babies, who have nostrils like dogs, and the haplorhines, who do not. And the haplorhines begat the tarsiers and the anthropoids. And these anthropoids begat the new world monkeys and the catarrhines, who have narrow nostrils facing downwards. And the cattarhines begat the old world monkeys and the hominoids, and the hominoids begat the gibbons and the great apes.

18. Behold, the great apes begat the orang-utan and the begetter of chimpanzees, gorillas and hominids. And then the begetter of gorillas departed from the begetter of chimpanzees and hominids. After this time, the begetter of chimpanzees also departed, and left the begetter of hominids alone.

19. And the begetter of hominids, said unto herself and unto her mate (for she could speak): let us beget more hominids. And they begat homo erectus who begat homo sapiens, which is to say humankind.

I have been trying to find a short contemporary narrative of human descent. As I could not, I decided to write one myself, in Biblical style. I will not be surprised if readers now inform me of other, similar versions already in existence. I have drawn on three sources: *The Variety of Life* by Colin Tudge [1], *The Ancestor's Tale* by Richard Dawkins [2] and the Tree of Life website [3]. Inevitably, only a tiny number of our ancestors or cousins, alive or extinct, are represented here. Some of the evolutionary lines are controversial. I have omitted others because they are unnamed or unknown. I hope that professional cladists will forgive me, even if scriptural fundamentalists do not.

1. Tudge C. *The Variety of Life: A Survey and a Celebration of All the Creatures That Have Ever Lived.* Oxford: Oxford University Press, 2000
2. Dawkins R. *The Ancestor's Tale.* London: Weidenfeld and Nicholson, 2005
3. The Tree of Life Project. *Tree of Life* http://tolweb.org/tree

14 The condition of music

Medicine and music are always jostling up against each other. Many medics are also keen amateur musicians. No doubt a sizeable proportion of the readers are flautists, fiddlers or singers, although I have to confess that I gave up the French horn after Grade Six following a family ultimatum. You may be aware of a number of notable musicians who first trained as doctors. The conductor Jeffrey Tate and the opera singer Emer McGilloway are current British examples.

It may be no coincidence that these two interests are so commonly shared. The worlds of music and of medicine may be related to each other, for reasons that we recognize intuitively but are hard put to describe in words. I took a step closer to understanding this at a conference in Cambridge on 'Narrative Based Medicine'. It was the end of the first morning, the presentations had overrun, and I badly wanted my lunch. I probably would have slipped out, but this meant walking directly past Professor Trisha Greenhalgh in the chair, and I was scared that she would glare at me disapprovingly. Because of this I stayed on for the final speaker, a philosopher called Martyn Evans. His topic, as it happened, was medicine as music.

Instead of starting his presentation immediately, he first played a recording of Bach – a piece from 'The Well Tempered Klavier'. The moment was spellbinding. I forgot my rumbling stomach. I would happily have missed my lunch – and indeed the whole afternoon – to hear all the 48 preludes and fugues in the book. I looked round at the hundreds of assembled doctors, researchers, teachers and social scientists, and they all seemed transported to a place that none of the preceding lectures (excellent as they all were) could possibly have taken them. When the music came to an end, it seemed hardly necessary for Professor Evans to say a word. However, he somehow managed to articulate what the piece itself had conveyed subliminally.

He spoke of how music creates narrative without representation. He suggested that music provides an organizing metaphor for medical practice. He argued that 'medicine belongs to music' as the imaginative creation of order amid chaos.

This claim rings true. Yet it also challenges us profoundly as doctors. On the one hand, we regard such models of medicine as entertaining, but cannot believe that they might be seen as a serious alternative to the application of reason. On the other hand, we recall our real-life encounters with patients, and we have to acknowledge that there are nearly always some processes going on that cannot be understood at all through reason. They are processes that remind us inescapably of rhythm, cadence, and the elaboration of themes towards a resolution.

The nineteenth century critic Walter Pater claimed that all art aspired to the condition of music. If medicine is an art, then it shares with its fellow arts that same yearning towards wordlessness, and towards communication through abstract aerial vibration alone. If you try to analyse why you took a medical history from a particular person in a particular way, or why you offered information with the exact nuance that you did, or why the patient ended up pursuing one treatment option rather than another, it may be impossible to understand these except in terms of an instinctive human capacity for composition. Unsettling as it is, it may be hard to resist the notion that science pays tribute to harmony, and not the other way round.

15 The professor of cheese

The most self-important person I have ever met was the proprietor of a cheese shop. He wasn't hostile, like the famous cheese salesman portrayed by John Cleese in the television sketch. He behaved more as if he was a professor of cheese studies at Oxbridge. If you named a cheese, he would hold forth on its history, its bacteriology, its merits and its drawbacks. He didn't sell Gorgonzola, only 'Mountain Gorgonzola'. I once asked him if he stocked valley Gorgonzola, but he didn't think that was funny. Then I had the temerity to ask for some 'cheap and cheerful Cheddar' for a cauliflower cheese. He explained solemnly that, if a cheese was worth cooking with, it was worth paying for, too.

We finally fell out when I arrived one day to find a hole in the pavement outside his shop, because a water main had burst. I asked him if one of his cheeses had exploded and he was furious. He had lost a lot of business that day because of the hole. I never dared to go in his shop again.

Looking back, I think my attempts to provoke him were rather ironic, since I probably belong to the most self-important profession of all. No one takes doctors more seriously than doctors themselves. Possibly this is because we lack any form of institutionalized court jester to take us down a peg or too. Unlike lawyers (at least until they become judges) we do not have opposing advocates trying to pick holes in every argument we propose. Unlike politicians, we do not have anyone to jeer at us, or throw eggs at our clean white coats. Our clients never tease us in the way I teased the cheese man. In day-to-day life, our self-importance goes largely unchallenged and therefore largely unexamined.

On the whole, the written literature of medicine only inflates our self-esteem even further. There are dozens of excellent books telling us how to become more compassionate and humane as doctors (and some hint subtly at the authors' eligibility for sainthood), but I cannot ever recall reading one that advised doctors to 'come off it!' This is a shame. The mentors who have most inspired me have shared a certain quality that I would describe as a twinkle. They knew when patients needed them to crack a joke or to swear. Above all, they seemed to take their patients far more seriously than they took themselves.

There is a corollary to this. Pomposity actually sits better on many other professions than it does on doctors. I have enjoyed many an evening out in good restaurants, admiring head waiters who knew how to play their part. They understood that their job required a certain sense of theatre, and a performance of gravitas, in order to make customers feel that they were getting their money's worth. Had they been cardiologists, their comportment would have been ludicrous. Medicine is too serious a job for acting a part. Patients need authenticity, and they can spot fake piety or defensive arrogance a mile off. Most would probably prefer their consultant to chuckle rather than to pontificate.

Shedding self-importance also conveys a further message: when all is said and done, medicine is just a job. Some people are road menders and some are hairdressers; it is a moot point whether doctors end up making people's lives safer or happier than these professions, or many others. We also become doctors for a variety of reasons that are no more moral or immoral than anyone else's reasons for choosing their occupation. Yet unlike others, we seem to buy into the delusion that we are special.

It really is a delusion. I remember when I first discovered this as a house physician. I walked onto the ward one evening carrying a portable ECG machine, but pretended I had brought some tools to mend the TV. The patients thought at first that I was serious, and were bitterly disappointed when they discovered I had neither the tools nor the skill to fix it.

When I say that medicine is 'just a job', it may seem dismissive or even contemptuous. I do not mean it in that way. I think we should reclaim the phrase as a token of proportionate humility. There is honour in ordinariness, and maybe sanity too. I sometimes wonder if the crimes of medical murderers such as Shipman and Bodkin Adams arose not just from some quirk of brain biochemistry or childhood deprivation, but also from an exaggerated sense of professional self-importance. In them, it may have been writ very large indeed, but it is never entirely absent in medical institutions. The collective conscience of the profession usually keeps it within bounds, but not always.

16 What's in a name?

I handed a prescription to a patient last week and she asked me whether she should take it straight away '*to the apothecary*'. I thought at first that she was using the word apothecary as a joke, but she was not. At the age of 97, she was saying it without any self-consciousness – and presumably without any awareness that dictionaries have defined it as archaic for at least 50 years.

I wondered if I was witnessing the very last time that this word would ever be used in common English parlance, apart from rarefied usages – as in the Society of Apothecaries. Doctors spend their lives listening to people, so we may be in a better position than almost anyone else to listen out for archaic words that have survived in common speech. Of course, it would be impossible scientifically – in the Popperian sense – to record the last usage of any word. Who could ever prove that the word 'milliner', or 'costermonger', or indeed 'apothecary' would never be spoken again?

To chronicle the very *first* usage of each word in the English language was, in its time, the biggest research project ever undertaken – the 19th century equivalent of the human genome project. A doctor, as it happens, played a large part in this. When James Murray began to compile the Oxford English Dictionary in 1879, he solicited the help of an army of enthusiastic volunteers from around Britain. He asked them to comb the published literature in the English tongue since mediaeval times, and to record examples of the first appearance of every English word, in each of its nuances. One of Murray's most prolific correspondents, particularly for words beginning with 'A' and 'B', was William Chester Minor, an American surgeon, resident in Berkshire.

Minor had more opportunity – and perhaps more motivation – to go about this task than one might expect from most surgeons. He was a traumatized survivor of the American civil war, a paranoid schizophrenic, a convicted murderer, and an inmate of Broadmoor Hospital. Writing from a comfortable suite of rooms in the hospital (financed from his US army pension), Minor religiously posted his carefully researched examples to Murray in his corrugated iron shed in Mill Hill. Over a period of 20 years, he sent in about 12 000 standardized slips. Murray was to write, 'So enormous have been Dr Minor's contributions ... that we could easily illustrate the last four centuries from his quotations alone.' Only in his later years, when he had cut off his own penis in a fit of post-masturbatory guilt, did Minor's offerings cease altogether. The entire poignant and bizarre story can be read in Simon Winchester's book *The Surgeon of Crowthorne*[1].

When my elderly patient used the word apothecary, I naturally asked her if she meant that she ought to take her prescription to the 'chemist'. I was then struck by an irony. I too had betrayed my age – because of course these days chemists do not exist either. They are known as pharmacists.

In superficial terms, apothecaries, chemists and pharmacists are all the same. They are all people who make up medicines and sell them. Yet at the same time, we also know that they are quite different creatures. Each title carries a different weight, and a different set of mental associations. Chemists wanted us to call them pharmacists because it sounded grander. The strategy has worked, and their job status has become enhanced as a result. When you change a word, you also affect the thing it denotes.

Many philosophers nowadays argue that language not only describes reality, it also creates it. The case of apothecaries, chemists and pharmacists is a fairly straightforward example of this process at work. As doctors, we can also note how some diseases have entirely vanished when we ceased to believe in their names (such as neurasthenia), while new names have been conjured into existence to explain the inexplicable (such as irritable bowel syndrome).

These examples of the creative power of language are fairly easy to accept, but there are some even bigger challenges to our basic professional assumptions. For example, there are compelling arguments to suggest that even words like 'asthma' or 'hypertension' each cover a particular constellation of symptoms, signs, treatments and aetiological explanations that may evaporate utterly over time. It is not just a question, say the philosophers, of having to hone down our diagnoses or explanatory theories about these conditions, so that they gradually become more accurate. Our whole systems of thought about disease may in fact be no more than a set of self-referential linguistic fabrications. This isn't something we can ever hope to change; it is inherent in the nature of language itself.

This idea may seem counter-intuitive, or even absurd. That may be simply because we think in language itself, so we believe uncritically in the reality it generates. In the same way, my patient believed she could still take her prescription to an apothecary.

1. Winchester S. *The Surgeon of Crowthorne, a tale of murder, madness and the love of words.* Penguin, 1999

17 A house divided

Hospital consultants and GPs are full of prejudices about each other. Generally, GPs envy hospital doctors – especially academic ones – as important people gifted with fierce intelligence, an unflinching focus, and encyclopaedic learning. Catch us at a jaded moment, however, and we may confess a mild contempt for them, as impossibly narrow-minded folk who cannot tell their proctalgia fugax from their lateral epicondylitis. In the same way, consultants probably think on the whole that we GPs are unimportant amateurs, but nevertheless will admit at times to feeling cowed by the broadness of our competence.

In reality, the main difference between GPs and specialists like physicians probably lies in our degree of preference for conceptual boundaries – something that may be determined by personality type. Unlike specialists, GPs need to possess a facility for tracking patients' lives and narratives across wildly varying terrain, heedless of the fences we have to leap over. In any one consultation, we may have to move between orthopaedics and psychiatry, biology and biography, and even between medicine, social work and theology. Not long ago, for example, I saw a mother and her two small children in my surgery. They felt pole-axed by the sudden and unexpected departure of the father from the home. At the end of the consultation I inquired if there was any important ground that we had not covered. The mother replied: 'Can you look in Jordan's ears to see if he's got any wax.' Of course I said yes.

It is reassuring to think that specialists and generalists complement each other by thinking in different ways. At the same time, we should not be led into believing that the distinction between the two species is unalterable. In his classic study, *The Division in British Medicine*[1], Frank Honigsbaum traced the historical process by which successive political interventions, together with intraprofessional prejudices, intensified the divide between hospital consultants and general practitioners in Britain during the twentieth century. He argued that the division – far sharper than in many other countries – not only impeded continuity of patient care but critically limited what the National Health Service could achieve.

I met Frank Honigsbaum a few years ago, and he was astonished to learn that I was both a GP and a part-time National Health Service consultant, since this seemed to contradict his thesis. Yet there are probably no more than a few dozen doctors like me in Britain with this dual identity. To the best of my knowledge, all our posts were created during a kind of collective panic among NHS trusts in the 1990s, after the Conservative government had offered GP practices their own budgets for purchasing secondary services. At that time, there was a marked – almost embarrassing – improvement in the way that hospital consultants spoke and wrote to GPs. Some of us were even appointed as 'consultants in general practice' in hospitals and elsewhere, hence my own post. Perceptions had changed.

In the event, many GPs thought that budgets were divisive, and fewer than half signed up for them. When a Labour government took over in 1997, it promised to transform the scheme into something far more equitable by bringing all GPs into commissioning agencies, in the form of primary care groups. One consequence of this was that our importance as a profession seemed assured.

Things turned out very differently. Primary care groups were all 'promoted' to trusts but, crucially, GPs were assigned only minority representation on them. It is hard to know whether this was a ruse that the government had intended all along, or a change of plan. Whatever the truth may have been, most GPs soon came to see the new organizations as instruments of centralized management and policing. We were not so important after all.

1. Honigsbaum F. *The Division in British Medicine: A History of the Separation of General Practice from Hospital Care, 1911–1968.* London, Palgrave Macmillan, 1979

18   Seeing double

I doubt that I have much in common with William Shakespeare or Margaret Thatcher. However, we do share one important bond – as parents of opposite-sex twins.

Once you have twins, you join one of those invisible networks of affinity that cut across class and culture. It is similar to the affinity that people discover when they share a particular medical condition, for example, or are immigrants. What unites you is the realization that no one – least of all professionals such as doctors – can fully understand that particular aspect of your life unless they have had the same experience. You also suddenly find yourself taking an intense interest in an aspect of the world to which you were previously quite indifferent.

Parents of twins all report one thing: twins are regarded as public property. As Anne Shakespeare wheeled Hamnet and Judith out in their oak baby carriage, you can be sure that the citizens of Stratford stopped her to inquire: *'Are they boys or girls?'*, *'Which is the dominant one?'*, *'Do they get on?'* Dennis Thatcher, on his expeditions with Carol and Mark in their Silver Cross perambulator, no doubt soon tired of scowling at people who pointed out: *'You've got your hands full!'* The phrase, with its asinine claim for originality, echoes endlessly in your ears. It usually sounds like a mixture of exorcism and envy.

Yet the phrase at least shows you that people understand the size of your task. Twins bring with them a merciless kind of arithmetic. With only one baby at a time, parents can take it in turns to go to the toilet unaccompanied. When you have twins, neither of you has this luxury. Both parents have to learn to do most things while carrying a child, unless someone else is willing to get stuck in too. The intrusiveness of strangers may in fact be an evolved response to your need for communal help.

The commonest question you face is, of course, *'Are they identical?'* The question has a kind of ritual, mantric quality, quite dissociated from any knowledge or understanding of zygosity. Even doctors have asked if our boy and girl are identical. ('No,' I sometimes answer, 'the boy has a penis.') Ignorance about the difference between monozygous (MZ) and dizygous (DZ) twins is almost universal. Contrary to obstetric myth, you cannot tell by looking at the placenta. The placenta of MZ twins can split into two, and DZ placentas can fuse. From intrauterine life, MZ twins can vary greatly in appearance – particularly in size – while same-sex DZ twins, like any siblings, can look like peas in a pod. At 20 weeks of gestation, the behaviour patterns of MZ twins, visible on ultrasound, can be as different from each other as any DZ pair. The only true standard for zygosity is DNA testing.

The frequency of twins in Britain, especially DZ twins, is increasing fast. This is partly because of the dramatically accelerated success rate in implanted embryos. It is also because women are having children when they are older – a factor that also increases the chances of twins. Twinhood is sensitive to other maternal parameters too. In the words of Elizabeth Bryan, the doyenne of twin studies in Britain, and co-founder of the Twins and Multiple Births Association, if you want to have twins 'it is best to be a six foot Nigerian in your late thirties who already has five children including a set of fraternal twins'.

Twins have always been common in literature. Not surprisingly, Shakespeare was himself fond of depicting them. The farcical plot in *The Comedy of Errors* revolves around two sets of twins, while in *Twelfth Night*, Sebastian and Viola are meant to look so similar that 'an apple cleft in twain is not more twin'. One of the greatest novels of recent years in English – *The God of Small Things* by Arundhati Roy – tells the story of opposite-sex twins, and of the consequences of their separation.

One story, perhaps more than any other, has influenced our perception of twins and how they relate to each other: that of Jacob and Esau. Most people can recall learning about their enmity, especially Jacob's extortion of his brother's inheritance for 'a mess of pottage', and his trickery in persuading their blind father Isaac to bless him, in the guise of his hairier sibling. However, the prolonged tale of their rivalry and estrangement, which extends over eight chapters of Genesis, ends in a moving reconciliation. After his long absence from Canaan, Jacob returns to meet his twin: 'And Esau ran to meet him, and embraced him, and fell on his neck, and kissed him: and they wept' (Genesis 33:4).

The reconciliation is so startling, and perhaps so challenging emotionally, that not all readers have accepted it at face value. The seventh century Massoretic editors of the Hebrew Bible, for example, indicated that the words 'he kissed him' could also be read as 'he bit him'. Whatever the reason for this – and many have been suggested – they captured the ambivalence that twins can show to each other, sometimes moving in a moment between fierce conflict and mutual generosity. And yet, since my wife and I became parents of twins and started to inquire about such things, we have scarcely ever met a twin who did not feel blessed to be one.

19 The art of questioning

A physician once saved my life with a question, or more precisely, with two questions.

I had been short of breath for several months. Because I had had some cardiac problems in the past – an episode of pericarditis seven years previously – I called my cardiologist. He thought it sounded like a slight worsening of my generally mild asthma, and reassured me. As the weeks passed, I had good days and bad days, and sometimes I worried more and sometimes less. At some point I organized a chest X-ray and an ECG for myself, and I also saw my GP. The tests were normal, there were no physical signs of anything, and the message was one of unconcerned uncertainty.

Then one day I could not walk to the shops at the end of the road without stopping. My wife thought that my lips were now slightly blue. She insisted that my GP should send me to hospital.

In the back of my mind I had a nagging fear that I was having pulmonary emboli. In any logical sense, this seemed absurd. I had no pain in my chest or legs, no cough and no haemoptysis. I was generally fit, and had not gone on any long flights that year. But my mother had died of a pulmonary embolus during a hospital admission. Also, for the first time in my life, I was unaccountably having dreams about her brother, who was murdered by the Nazis as a teenager – almost certainly by cyanide asphyxiation in Auschwitz. I had not known him, and she had virtually never talked about him.

I saw a consultant chest physician who could not have been more thorough, but it was clear from her questions that pulmonary emboli did not figure remotely in her thinking. All the same, when she had finished examining me, she asked: 'Have you come up with any diagnosis yourself?' Sheepishly, and with the slight fear of ridicule that comes with not being a specialist, I told her of my specific anxiety. She then asked one further question: 'Does that mean you'd like a V/Q scan to reassure you?' I said yes. Three days later it was done, and showed I had already lost 25% of my lungs to multiple infarcts. 'You're a very good diagnostician' she said, graciously. I never told her about the bad dreams.

At medical school, we are taught meticulously about the importance of asking the right questions. Yet in our subsequent careers we often forget two of the most crucial ones: *'What do you think you've got?'* and *'How can I persuade you otherwise?'* As my physician demonstrated, the art of questioning clearly needs to go beyond the dry litany of formal history-taking and should embrace the patient's view as well. When we remember this, we nearly always save our patients many sleepless nights, and sometimes we save their lives too. (Even patients who are not medics can have improbable but correct intuitions about what is wrong with them.)

The art of questioning may go further still. One of the most challenging researchers ever to have looked at questions in clinical consultations is the Canadian psychologist Karl Tomm. He talks of conversations between professionals and patients as being treatments in themselves. He doesn't mean this in the relatively banal sense of offering reassurance or empathy. Instead he talks about 'questions as interventions' and of consultations as 'interventive interviewing'. He suggests that the chief purpose of clinical questioning is not primarily to pin problems down, but to try and redefine and resolve them through the conversational process itself. Although Tomm is writing principally about consultations in mental health settings, his approach to questioning may have equal, if not greater, application to medical contexts.

As a result of his researches, Tomm has proposed ways of using questions in order to call forth new and unexpected expressions, memories and ideas from the patient – including ones that they might otherwise not have expressed, or even thought. He makes a distinction between four principal types of questions. 'Lineal' questions are straightforward ones about facts and causes, the kind that doctors are asking all the time (*'how much alcohol do you drink?'*). 'Circular' questions invite people to think about themselves not as mere passive objects but as participants in a dynamic dance of human interactions (*'who gets most upset about your level of drinking?'*). 'Strategic' questions implicitly propose options for changing the situation (*'what help would you need if you tried to cut down on your drinking?'*). 'Reflexive' questions jolt patients into new ways of looking at their predicaments by examining them in an unexpected light (*'if you succeeded in giving up, are there other more difficult problems you might have to face?'*). Tomm counsels moving between these four types of questions, so that consultations are challenging without being confrontational, and never fall back into ritual or repetitiveness. One way of describing the kind of clinical interview that he teaches is as 'consultations inviting change'.

Tomm's original paper on questions has a stupefyingly off-putting title and it appears in a journal that few doctors will have heard of [1]. Nevertheless, I would say that it has influenced my professional behaviour more than anything I have ever read – and almost as much as the two questions that my chest physician asked.

1. Tomm K. Interventive interviewing: part III. Intending to ask lineal, circular, strategic or reflexive questions? *Family Process* 1988; **27**:1–15

20 Rhythms of life

Without a doubt, the school teacher who had the most profound effect on me was my sixth form English teacher. He had the ability to excite enthusiasm for the kind of knowledge that at first seems innately boring. So I came away from his lessons with, among other things, a lifelong fascination with poetic metre and rhythm.

Metre and rhythm, he taught, are not the same. Metre is the implacable drum beat that underlies any piece of verse (excepting some modern poetry). Rhythm is the actual pattern of conversational stress that you hear when the verse is spoken aloud. Sometimes the two coincide, but when they do not, the effect can be striking. To give an obvious example, the metre that lies behind most Shakespearean verse is as follows:

Ti TUM ti TUM ti TUM ti TUM ti TUM

If metre and rhythm were always the same, Shakespeare's most famous line would therefore go:

To BE or NOT to BE, that IS the QUEST.

Instead, what Hamlet says is this:

To BE or NOT to BE, THAT is the QUEStion.

Consciously or unconsciously, our attention is arrested by the premature fourth stress, and by the weak extra syllable at the end. There is an almost shocking disjunction between what our minds anticipate and what our ears hear. It is this tension between the expected and the observed, the confluence of altered arithmetic with altered meaning, that creates the drama of poetry and distinguishes inspiration from platitude. Of course, exactly the same thing is true in medicine.

There is another analogy worth pointing out between poetry and medicine. The favoured metre of English poetry – iambic pentameter – exactly reproduces normal human heart sounds, counted on the five fingers of one hand:

Lup DUP lup DUP lup DUP lup DUP lup DUP.

(Next time you listen to a healthy heart, try reciting 'Shall I compare thee to a summer's day?' while counting your fingers at the same time, and you will see what I mean – although it may take some explaining to the patient.) The effect in the line from Hamlet can therefore be likened quite accurately to the sense of subliminal unease that attends a ventricular extrasystole. Other, more elaborate effects mimic more sinister dysrhythmias. Thus King Lear's dying, disjointed words decelerate progressively into asystole:

Do you see this? Look on her, look, her lips,
Look there, look there!

It would be nice to think that this likeness between poetry and cardiology could be applied universally. Sadly it cannot. While some other languages such as French and Russian often trot along in iambic metres like English, others do not. Classical Greek verse gallops along on trisyllabic hooves, sounding to our ears alarmingly like an imitation of heart failure. Sanskrit and Hebrew metres flutter and fibrillate, with varying numbers of syllables between each stress. It is tempting to pathologize other cultures while seeing one's own as the epitome of health. However, it is probably more scientific to recognise that it is just a nice coincidence that English metre usually resembles a healthy heart, so that our poetic rhythms can be understood through cardiac metaphors.

It is also worth remembering that the distinction between poetry and prose is, in any case, a somewhat artificial one. Poetic rhythms can diverge so far from any recognizable metre that they turn into 'free verse'. Conversely, prose can become raised to the density and regularity of poetry. Remarkably, researchers in Glasgow have noticed that the latter phenomenon occurs in the speech of terminally ill patients, and they have demonstrated this by writing out some of their patient's stories in verse [1]. The following stanza comes from a recording they made of a lung cancer sufferer, as he describes the moment his consultant told him the diagnosis:

He said
'Well,'
He said,
'I'm not going
To beat about the bush'
He said
'You've got
A tumour in there
And a blockage,
And it's cancerous'
He didn't mess
He just told me
There and then.

These lines are not so much Shakespearean as biblical. With their short, irregular rhythms and their bleak, unremitting refrain of 'he said', they echo the poetry of the prophets, as transmitted firstly into the Latin Vulgate by St Jerome, and thence into English by William Tyndale and the great Jacobean translators.

Literary critics tell us that no text is ever entirely original; knowingly or not, each one refers back to prior texts and a prior tradition – a process known as intertextuality. So from the mouth of this dying Glaswegian we hear the unflinching directness of a Jeremiah or an Ezekiel. Perhaps if we listen to our patients carefully when they speak to us in clinics and on the wards, we may also hear echoes of Milton, Homer, the Mahabharata or the Epic of Gilgamesh.

1. Murray S, Kendall M, Boyd K et al. 'I knew ...' *Br J Gen Pract* 2001; **51**:776–7

21 Interpreting illness

The first piece of research I ever did was a study of interpreters. I did it during a student elective in northern Nigeria, with a Medical Research Council grant that paid my fare (just). I made audiotapes of out-patient consultations between patients who spoke Hausa and doctors who spoke English but used non-medical staff as interpreters. Once I had made the tapes, I asked some local medical students, all perfectly bilingual, to listen to them and translate all the Hausa statements. I looked at what the patients had actually said and then compared this with what was transmitted by the interpreters.[1]

Not surprisingly, I found all sorts of deviations between the patients' utterances and what the interpreters conveyed. Some of these deviations were quite legitimate. For example, skilled staff could run through part of a systems inquiry on their own initiative and then report, quite accurately: 'His urine's normal' or 'He doesn't have any breathing problems'. On the other hand, I discovered some alarming errors, where interpreters had reported that the patients had said something they had not. Also, the interpreters were pretty selective in what they wanted the doctor to know, and occasionally they even berated patients for apparent inconsistencies.

I wrote some guidelines for using interpreters, based on what I found. They went as follows (please excuse the sexist language – it was the 1970s): 'Greet the patient to establish direct contact. Be seen to be in charge of the interpreter. Assess the interpreter's English and try to find out how well he speaks the patient's language. Assess his interests: he may be an anxious relative or an indifferent auxiliary. Give only short sentences for translation, and get the interpreter to explain that the patient must do the same. Make sure everything is translated. Check every answer by asking questions in two or three ways. Finally, use the interpreter to tell the patient everything you would tell him if he could speak your language.'

Nearly 25 years later I would stand by a few of these rubrics, especially the first and last. But I would recant most of the others. Through experience of using interpreters a great deal myself, I have lost my conviction in what one might call the more obsessive, even dictatorial parts of this guidance. Nowadays it seems to me that the presence of an interpreter, whether in person or by phone link, radically changes the nature of a medical encounter, so that it may be an error to try and force it to resemble something it is not – a one-to-one conversation in a single language. I have even come to think that using interpreters may teach us something important about the nature of all medical encounters and how to conduct them.

I have noticed, for example, that patients speaking in their own language do not like to have their narrative flow interrupted for translation, even when the doctor believes that this needs to happen for diagnostic or therapeutic reasons. To put it at its simplest, it appears that patients want quite literally to be *heard*, and they may care relatively little whether the main hearer is someone with medical skills or not. I have also noticed that most interpreters, whether they are close relatives of the patient or paid professionals, have personal resources that go beyond the skill of literal, word-for-word, translation. They usually bring to the conversation a welcome freight of shared cultural associations, and thus an ability to contextualize utterances that might otherwise evaporate into meaninglessness. Such resources, of course, give the lie to the notion that 'pure' translation actually exists, independent of deeper interpretation – a delusion that no professional literary translator would ever suffer from.

As I have become aware of these things, I have gradually learned to sit back and to watch with respect as consultations of apparent intensity and effectiveness unfold between patient and interpreter in spite of – or because of – my passivity. For several minutes at a time, I remain content to understand very little, at least in the linguistic sense. I do this particularly with interpreters whom I have used on many occasions before, and have learned to trust. In such instances, I follow one principle only, asking myself: 'How little do I need to understand, to be confident that no harm is being done here?'. That aside, I take the risk of believing that the exchange is serving the purpose that the patient needs, and I try to suppress a wish to intrude my own professional purposes instead.

I suspect that many of my medical colleagues may feel uncomfortable with this confession. Equally, I have no doubt that many anthropologists and sociologists would strongly approve. Much contemporary social science research shows how we as doctors are being naïve when we imagine that patients tell us their histories chiefly so that we can formulate an accurate diagnosis or recommend a treatment. These are usually our main preoccupations, but they may not be the patient's. Illness narratives serve far wider, and perhaps far more urgent and essential purposes. For example, they allow patients, through the very act of speaking, to fashion their memories and sensations into a coherent shape. They provide people with opportunities to assign causation, purpose and direction to their experiences, and to claim moral legitimacy for their own actions.[2] Like all personal narratives, they enable people to describe who they are, discover who they are becoming, and define who they wish to be.[3]

Telling a story to another person about one's experiences is the principal way of locating the self, perhaps even of constructing it. For such a task, it may be that an interpreter is at least as good a collaborator as a doctor, and may be considerably better. Perhaps we should all have interpreters present when we visit our physicians.

1. Launer J. Taking medical histories through interpreters: practice in a Nigerian outpatient department. *Br Med J* 1978; **2**:934–5.
2. Bury M. Illness narratives: fact or fiction? *Soc Health Illn* 2001; **23**:263–85.
3. Mattingly C. *Healing Dramas and Clinical Plots: The Narrative Structure of Experience*. Cambridge University Press, Cambridge, 1998.

22   Close encounters

I am sometimes asked to run seminars on primary care for other professions, particularly social workers and psychologists. Like some hospital doctors, people in these professions can have odd ideas of what primary care is and does, and even odder stereotypes about GPs. One of the ways I tackle these stereotypes is to ask seminar members to get into pairs and tell each other about recent encounters with GPs. I ask them to exchange one story about a professional encounter, followed by one story about a personal encounter when they have visited GPs' surgeries as patients, carers or parents.

A striking contrast often emerges between the two sets of stories. Tales of professional encounters usually centre on the frustrations of trying to contact GPs during busy surgeries, or the mutual incomprehension that can occur when trying to discuss a case or elicit some information from a GP. The personal stories, on the other hand, generally have quite a different tone. They speak of longstanding, trusting and even tender relationships with family doctors. They testify to people's capacity to tolerate all the huge and conspicuous inadequacies of general practice in exchange for the things they value: a listening ear, a warm touch, some blunt advice, and the ability to display friendliness without an inappropriate claim to friendship. This contrast can lead people to hold a subtler and less edgy view of primary care.

However, there is another exercise that is even more fruitful in this respect. It is to ask people to share memories of the GPs they saw when they were children. Childhood memories of family doctors can be very powerful, and it is unfair to set this exercise without being prepared to reflect on one's own recollections. And so I find myself casting my mind back to the three GPs of my own childhood and adolescence: Dr Newman, Dr Tanner, and Dr Dean.

Dr Newman was a refugee from Nazi Germany. We used to go into his consulting room from the waiting room when a red light came on, but afterwards we went out straight through the back door into his yard, so you never knew how much time he spent alone between patients. Sometimes he asked you how many people there still were in the waiting room. My mother came from Vienna – in the same era and for the same reason – so they spoke together in German. Dr Newman dispensed lots of practical advice, and once told my mother to go out and buy a fridge, which she did. He was famous in our family for always claiming to suffer from whatever ailment you came with. '*Das hab ich auch!*' he would say: '*I've got that too!*' The favourite family story about him (a myth perhaps, who knows?) was about the day my mother went to him with a foot complaint. He took off his shoes and socks, and then put his feet up on the desk to prove his claim. After that, we changed our doctor. As an adult, I can guess at the reasons why his relentless claims for sympathy for his own suffering became intolerable for my mother.

We moved to Dr Tanner. For some reason I am entirely unable to explain, I am quite certain she was a Roman Catholic. She was very well spoken, and there was an aura about her that she was 'a cut above' the area of London where we lived and she practised. (How can a child of two continental refugees have been so aware of English accents, religious denominations and class? Yet it seems I was.) She was frail-looking, tense and pale, and I connect that in my mind with her departure after only three or four years, although that connection may only be a fantasy.

She was replaced by Dr Dean, whose most striking feature to a nine-year-old boy was the prodigious quantity of hair growing from his ears. He was Indian, and my adult self deduces that he was a Sikh, although he did not wear a turban. One of the most magical things he used to do was to reach into the drawers of his desk for samples of ointments that visiting reps had just left for him. He would then hand them over to my mother to try out on my eczema. As a result, I tried out topical steroids for the first time. Hence I was able to throw away the thick tar ointments that had befouled my bedclothes for years, and the bandages I had had to wear under my trousers at school. I loved the presence, smell and feel of Dr Dean: burly, squidgy and comforting all at the same time. The last time I saw him was in late adolescence for a medical before I went off to teach in Kenya for my gap year. I was convinced he was going to discover the extensive cancer I had been concealing for years. He didn't, and so my trip went ahead. On my return from Africa, I went to a university doctor who told me my fears were ungrounded. I had been suffering all through my teens from widespread lymphadenopathy as the consequence of my eczema.

I have no idea if these three numinous figures influenced my eventual decision (halfway through university) to become a doctor and then a GP. But I recognize in these memories – and the memories evoked in my seminars – a truth that we often ignore or forget. The experience that patients have of doctors is quintessentially a sensual, affective and aesthetic one. Moral and cognitive judgements may displace our consciousness of this, but they cannot obliterate it. At the core of all our professional encounters, the acuity of childhood still persists.

23 All doctors are liars

Probably the best way to stop doctors from reading anything is to use the word 'postmodernism'. Assuming you are still reading, however, I will try to give an account of postmodernism, and why I think every doctor needs to understand it.

Postmodernism isn't a single theory. It's more of an attitude that governs many people's thinking nowadays. The reason that postmodernism goes by that name is that it rejects the 'modern' claim that we can discover increasingly better truths about the world. Instead, it argues that all we can do is continually to produce different ones, each reflecting our own historical, political and cultural perspectives. All knowledge, say postmodernists, is perspectival.

Postmodernism challenges the authority of all the big traditional bodies of knowledge like science and medicine. It also challenges other bodies of knowledge that you may or may not care about, like Marxism and psychoanalysis. According to postmodernism, these are all just 'grand narratives' – in other words, jolly good stories that a lot of people have agreed to believe for a period of time, but stories nevertheless. The only difference between these and fiction, say postmodernists, is that there are more people around who have decided to believe in the second law of thermodynamics, the Krebs cycle, progress, or the unconscious mind, than in Goldilocks and the three bears.

Now you may just sigh with exasperation and decide that only the French could come up with such silly ideas. (And it was the French – at least initially. Famous names involved include Foucault, Derrida and Lyotard.) However, it is worth remembering that all knowledge does indeed have a sell-by date. Typical examples in medicine are the many 'diseases' like neurasthenia, which have ceased to be something that anyone believes in, or even bothers to try and understand, or remember. Or you can think on a bigger scale, and imagine what the ancient Egyptians, the Sumerians or the Minoans would have thought if anyone had told them that their systems of medicine, and indeed their whole ways of understanding the world, would one day be entirely meaningless. Then project yourself forward in your imagination, and it is not hard to conceive of a world in the far future where people unearth a copy of *Gray's Anatomy* and shake their heads in astonishment at the way we saw things. If indeed they think of themselves as having heads.

There are two very obvious objections to postmodernism, and you may already have thought of them. One is that postmodernism is 'a claim to know truth that challenges all claims to know truth' and therefore it seems to disqualify itself. In philosophical terms, this is similar to Epimenides' paradox. (Epimenides was the annoying Cretan who used to go around saying that all Cretans were liars.) Postmodernists respond to this objection by invoking irony. They point out that every statement that anyone ever makes should carry the self-effacing rider: '*But of course I'm only saying this because of who I am...*'. Their defence is that at least postmodernists are saying this openly. In other words, postmodernism supplies its own ironic nudge and wink, and urges us all to do the same.

The other obvious objection to postmodernism is along the lines of: 'If you kick postmodernists, I bet they get bruises like everyone else.' It can be very tempting to kick postmodernists and they do indeed get bruises, but I need to warn you that when they pick themselves off the ground they are liable to argue something like this: '*I only got a bruise because, from my current perspective, I cannot yet imagine a world where something different happens.*'

If you aren't yet tearing your hair out, I have some good news for you. There are 'hard' postmodernists, so to speak, but there are also 'soft' ones. Hard postmodernists will go on talking about perspectival knowledge even when you threaten to batter them to death, and if you are exceptionally unlucky, they will mutter something about death being only a cultural construction, as they expire. Soft postmodernists, however, will eventually say '*It's a fair cop!*' They will admit that some kind of reality probably does exist 'out there', even though they will still try to convince you that most of the claims you make about it are irredeemably infused with subjectivity, vested interests and special pleading.

The reason that postmodernism matters to doctors is this. While 'hard' postmodernism has had very little influence outside the rarefied worlds of academic philosophy and social science, 'soft' postmodernism has had a huge public influence. It has changed people's conceptual landscapes irrevocably. To put it bluntly, fewer and fewer people think that we as doctors can offer them 'the truth'. Increasingly, they believe that we are offering them one kind of truth among many available. Whether their perspectives are informed by consumerism, complementary medicine, feminism, multiculturalism, opposition to multinationals, or any of the other hundreds of streams of contemporary thought, the patients who sit in our waiting rooms are no longer likely to accept that the scientific and medical views of the world trump all others. They are, in effect, soft postmodernists.

As far as they are concerned, everything we say is prefaced by the phrase: '*But of course I'm only saying this because I'm a doctor...*' Perhaps we would do better to say it ourselves.

24 Mentioned in passing

For over twenty years, my main place of work was in Edmonton. As London suburbs go, Edmonton is definitely not chic. Some Londoners have never even heard of it. Others only know it as the place where most of London's garbage is incinerated. Most simply have a vague impression of it as somewhere that flashes by on the North Circular Road, or on the A10 to Cambridge. Essentially, Edmonton is on the way from somewhere to somewhere else.

Edmonton is transitional in other ways too. Few of our patients were actually born here. Even fewer dream of living out the rest of their days in Edmonton. Some have moved here from Hackney or Tottenham in order to buy their first property, and now their greatest hope is to move out of London altogether, to the leafy vales of Broxbourne or Waltham Abbey. Others have arrived as asylum seekers, but once they know London better, they have no wish to stay in Edmonton any more than they want to return to Kosovo, Somalia or Kurdistan. For them too, Edmonton is a staging post.

Perhaps it is no coincidence that Edmonton was once a staging post in a quite literal sense. Before the railway came, turning Edmonton from a pretty Middlesex village into a characterless London suburb, the stage coaches stopped here on their way out of the city and into Hertfordshire. Ironically, many Londoners over the centuries must have taken their first breath of country air around Edmonton Green.

Back in its village days, Edmonton had many literary connections, especially around the turn of the nineteenth century. Curiously, nearly all of these are of medical or psychiatric interest. One of Britain's most popular poets, John Keats, was apprenticed to a Dr Hammond in Church Street. Keats never completed his training, and later he moved to Hampstead. Nevertheless, on the site of Hammond's surgery there is now a Keats Parade with a Keats Pharmacy. Nearby, there is a Keats Surgery. The North Middlesex Hospital, which squats like a carbuncle on the North Circular Road, boasts a Keats Ward. Keats could hardly complain we have forgotten him.

Keats is not Church Street's only literary figure from that time. In the churchyard itself is the grave of Charles Lamb and his sister Mary – known to generations of children as the authors of 'Tales from Shakespeare'. Their original reason for leaving London was that Mary had murdered their mother while in the grip of delusions. Astonishingly for the time, she was not incarcerated, but allowed to stay in the care of her brother. They first moved to Enfield, but then came to Edmonton to obtain medical treatment for Mary's worsening schizophrenia. Alas, the task of being her carer told on Charles. He took to the bottle, and eventually died from the consequences of a fall. Mary never again recovered her sanity.

As well as figuring in these literary lives, Edmonton appears in one of England's best known comic poems: the ballad of John Gilpin. The ballad tells of a luckless London merchant who wanted to join his family at the Bell Inn in Edmonton, in order to celebrate his wedding anniversary. The celebration never happens. Through a farcical series of frights and mishaps, Gilpin is unable to stop his horse galloping past Edmonton into Hertfordshire, and then galloping straight back into London. The ballad is obviously poking fun at its hero, but could it be making a point about Edmonton as well? One is left wondering what is it about the place that has this effect on bipeds and quadrupeds alike.

The ballad's author, William Cowper, was never a resident of Edmonton, but he must have known it well as a passing place. He has since been adopted as an honorary Edmontonian: the Bell was renamed the John Gilpin Bell, and there is now a John Gilpin Ward at the 'North Midd' too.

Cowper himself led a life in many ways similar to Mary Lamb's. He spent most of it in the grip of a terrifying depressive psychosis. Like Mary Lamb, he had a devoted carer for many years – in his case, a widowed woman friend called Mrs Unwin. He too sank into permanent despair once his carer died. Before that, he wrote some of the most poignant descriptions we have of melancholy and paranoia. In his letters, Cowper explained that he wrote John Gilpin and many of his other poems in order to keep insanity at bay. He translated the whole of Homer not once but twice, doing a certain number of verses each day to fend off 'Mr Bluedevil'.

Unlike Keats, Cowper is no longer popular. You can go into just about any second-hand book shop in the country and pick up a long-discarded volume of his verse for fifty pence. Sadly it is unlikely to include his Homer, which is a masterpiece, and possibly the greatest of all the English translations. (His Iliad is out of print, but his Odyssey is still available in the Everyman edition.) I would take Cowper's complete works to my desert island in preference to Keats's poetry any day. But then I have always rebelled against fashion – which is probably why I still have a soft spot for Edmonton after all these years.

25 The National Illness Service

A few months ago, I had a conversation with a hospital chief executive who was complaining about the unrealistic expectations that many patients have nowadays. He told me that he wished we could change the name of the National Health Service to the National 'Keeping-Death-at-Bay' Service. He thought that this would help patients to shed their illusions of omnipotence and immortality. It would also indicate that, in reality, hospitals by themselves have little to do with the production of health.

This struck me as an interesting if somewhat provocative idea. However, I didn't give it much thought until the following month, when I happened to be doing some consultancy work for a mental health team in the south of England. During the course of this, the team leader said how much he disliked being part of something called a 'mental health team'. He thought this name was quite dishonest and really they ought to be called the 'Coping-With-Disappointment' team. After all, he argued, most of the patients they saw were simply struggling to come to terms with lives that had failed to fulfil their hopes. He and his colleagues could usually do little to alter this – but they could still do good work if people were inclined to accept that disappointment is inherent in the human condition.

When you come across an idea like this twice in quick succession, you can be pretty sure that you will soon come across it a third time. So when a friend recently recommended a book called '*How to be a good enough GP*',[1] I wasn't very surprised to find that it addressed exactly this theme, and elaborated it at some length.

The author of the book, Gerhard Wilke, is a social anthropologist and group analyst who has done a great deal of work with groups of GPs in the last few years, trying to help them to adjust to the numerous reforms and reorganizations that have unsettled doctors' lives so much in Britain. Wilke's book makes sense of a great deal that is going on in primary care at the moment, but I have no doubt that it will also make sense for other doctors too.

Wilke takes his title from the concept of the 'good enough mother', a term coined by D.W. Winnicott to describe mothers who can help their infants to face the emotional challenges of the real world, with confidence and trust. By analogy, a 'good enough' doctor is one who helps patients do the same. Wilke argues that the very same ability is also needed by managers if they want to help doctors with their daily work. Here are some examples of what Wilke says on this subject:

'I would suggest that it is necessary to challenge the implicit ideology underpinning such buzzwords as health, team, modernisation, accreditation and audit. The emphasis on health at the exclusion of illness is a denial of a large part of reality of primary care.'

'Healthcare professionals like to think positively as it is too unbearable to stay in touch with the inevitability of decline and death. It is hard to live with the awareness that general practice can do a lot for patients but ultimately it manages the process of patients finding a good enough death …'.

'Professionals need to create a more balanced discussion in which the emphasis on health is matched by a focus on death and chronic decline. Only when that is politically acceptable will we have a more honest and realistic debate about resources.'

I believe that Wilke is right when he criticizes the rhetoric that has possessed British health service management in the last decade, and when he draws attention to what underlies this, namely a fear of mortality. Reading the book has certainly deepened my own understanding of why my in-tray is brimming every day with those dreadful, neo-Stalinist reports from government agencies and local trusts, full of frothy optimism and photos of multi-ethnic staff groups, all smiling joyfully. It has also helped me to understand the inevitable counterpart to all this managerial mania: widespread demoralization among health professionals and even, in some places, despair.

But I believe Wilke is right too when he points out that as doctors we play an important part in this process. The whole charade of cheerfulness in which we are now caught up both mocks and exploits our own tendency to certain forms of psychological avoidance. It may even echo the reason why we became doctors in the first place, and maybe that is why we find it so hard to confront the charade. Wilke offers us a challenge by suggesting that we will only become 'good enough' doctors when we acknowledge that there is a fundamental deception at the heart of the National 'Health' Service, and that we are both its perpetrators and its victims.

1.   Wilke G. *How to be a Good Enough GP: Surviving and Thriving in the New Primary Care Organisations.* Oxford, Radcliffe Medical Press, 2002.

26 All Greek to me

The consultation was difficult from the start. The patient appeared to speak some English, but it was barely adequate. She had come into my surgery clutching two pieces of paper. She opened the first, which was a calendar of the past year. There were circles around almost every date, some in red biro and others in black. Some of the dates were annotated in her handwriting, in her native Greek. She was evidently trying to tell me about her periods. They were too long or too short, too frequent or not frequent enough – I was not sure which. I wondered if she was trying to get pregnant, or perhaps trying not to get pregnant. So far, it was hard to know.

She opened the second piece of paper. It was a picture from a pelvic ultrasound. I thought I could make out the uterus and a right-sided ovarian cyst (no great technical feat here, as they were labelled in English, for some reason). The cyst looked as if it was probably a fairly small and innocent one, maybe a corpus luteum cyst, but I was very far from certain.

She was flustered. She wanted to explain lots of things to me, and I guessed that she probably wanted me to explain lots of things to her too. She hadn't let us know in advance that she might need a lot of time or someone to translate. Reluctantly, I phoned through to the office and asked them to get a Greek interpreter on the line. By the time the call came through I was already running late, and I knew that my decision would make the whole session, and my mood, bloody.

Having a phone interpreter made things better, but not hugely. At least we managed to establish that the woman's periods were infrequent but prolonged. Also she had no wish to get pregnant, and she gasped with horror when the interpreter explained that I hadn't been sure. Apart from that, the story got more confused.

Through the interpreter, she explained that she was sure it was the cyst that was making her periods too long. A professor of gynaecology in Athens had told her so. Every time she had a long period, she explained, he used to give her injections of antibiotics to bring it to an end. There ought to be a word for the stories that patients tell about their previous encounters with doctors, especially the very common kind like this that have no perceptible relationship to recognizable diseases or familiar treatments, and that pile up 'non sequiturs' nightmarishly on each other. I wasn't sure whether (a) the patient had misunderstood what happened in Greece, (b) the doctor there was a quack, or (c) there was something I didn't know about single cysts, prolonged periods and antibiotics. I got even hotter under the collar at the thought of trying to unscramble the rapidly escalating muddle.

There are consultations that go very well and harmoniously and leave you with a nice warm feeling about what a caring and attentive doctor you are. There are other consultations where you wonder why you chose medicine as a career. Suddenly, you recall all those trivial and arbitrary circumstances that led to such apparent inevitability, and you find your mind wandering to all the paths in your life that you never took: novelist, traveller, philanderer, tycoon. Fighting off such thoughts with diminishing success, I tried desperately to ask a few more questions through the interpreter to establish even the most tenuous commonality between this woman's understanding and mine. Each question failed. Each answer seemed to open up a new and previously unimagined conceptual chasm.

Reader, I lost it. I stopped remotely trying to understand her problem, let alone to solve it. Instead, I hectored her (it certainly felt to me like hectoring) about the impossibility of dealing with complex problems in haste. I reproached her (it certainly felt like a reproach) with giving me inadequate notice of the time and facilities that would be needed. I confronted her (it certainly felt like a confrontation) with the fact that much of her story seemed either incomprehensible or implausible to me. I rounded off this tirade (it certainly felt like a tirade) by pointing out that I wasn't her regular doctor anyway and it would make far more sense to book next time with the doctor who knew her best, giving enough notice to the receptionists and so on and so forth...

I knew already that this was the kind of consultation that would later leave me wincing with secret shame at the recollection of my unprofessionalism towards this patient, let alone the appalling impression I must have created on the interpreter. This was certainly not an encounter that I could ever report to colleagues, let alone commit to print. And so it would no doubt have remained, had it not been for her response: *'You have been very kind, doctor, and I should like to see you next time.'*

I was speechless. I would certainly not have named kindness among the emotions I had been struggling with during the previous twenty minutes. How on earth could she have perceived me as kind? Perhaps she been struck by my willingness, albeit grudgingly, to call in the aid of an interpreter. Maybe she experienced my prolonged ranting at her about resources as entirely proportionate to the scale of her need. Or was she responding to something rather more intangible?

Time and again, we have to re-learn in this job that what patients seem to value in us is not usually technical expertise and certainly not charm. It may be the thing that we fear the most: being ourselves.

27 It takes two

In recent months I have spent quite a lot of time thinking, teaching and writing about supervision. Like most people who have been drawn towards the subject, I have become fascinated by the way that supervision lies at the intersection of clinical knowledge and self-awareness, and by the opportunities that it offers for both technical and ethical development.

The word 'supervision', I have found, is not at all straightforward. If you move among mental health professionals like counsellors and psychologists, for example, you will hear them use the word constantly and fairly casually. '*I must get some supervision on a tricky case that I'm seeing*', they say, or: '*I'm feeling a bit stuck – would you mind giving me a bit of supervision later?*' They may be asking for an extended conversation about a case, but equally they may be wanting no more than five minutes' chat over lunch. Used in this way, the word seems to carry no special sense of hierarchy or judgementalism, and no particular sense of formality either. Basically, supervision here means a bit of reflective time, of whatever length, to open up new ideas.

Doctors, by contrast, often seem rather allergic to the word 'supervision'. Until recently, we tended to avoid the word altogether as a profession, preferring more neutral terms like case discussion. Even now, many of my colleagues tell me that the idea of supervision smacks to them of something bossy and critical, and of telling people how to do their jobs – like a manager standing over someone at a supermarket till. This state of affairs is of course changing, and medics are now beginning to think of supervision in a similar way to other professions: not as having someone looking over your shoulder but as having someone looking after you. Nevertheless, my experience of teaching supervision to doctors is that, even when they manage to shake off their worries about being bossed about, they still think of supervision in terms of being given the 'right answers' to any problem rather than being invited to think about their work in an entirely different way – as a collaborative enterprise rather than an individualistic one.

What I have learned from mental health professionals – and now attempt to teach to doctors – is that supervision is not a teaching technique but essentially a state of mind. It is a state of mind in which both parties (supervisor and supervisee) implicitly acknowledge the limitations that arise whenever individuals see cases on their own. These limitations can affect us not just in the occasional case that seems to go badly wrong, but also in the generality of cases that seem to be going entirely right, but may only take on that appearance because we have become so excessively comfortable with ourselves.

When I see a patient by myself, for example, I am limited not just by the boundaries of my experience and my knowledge base, but also by the fact that I am who I am. I can often make up for the limitations of my experience and knowledge quite easily by using a textbook or the internet, or by the simple expedient of knocking on someone's door and asking them a straightforward question. However, the limitations that arise from being myself are inescapable. All the questions I can think of asking the patient, and all the formulations I can think of about the case, simply cannot burst forth from the inevitable rigidities of self. Nor will any amount of training ever alter this fact. The only thing that can effectively change my thinking about any case is an encounter with another person who is able to interrogate my certainties, and perturb me into the vertiginous experience of remembering (yet again) that reality always can be seen from many different perspectives.

The task of clinical supervision, seen in this light, is not principally to explore the gaps in a colleague's knowledge, nor to propose alternative actions. It is a more philosophical task: namely, to detect and inquire into any automatic and unexamined habits of thinking and feeling. Whether one is supervising a psychoanalyst or an orthopaedic surgeon, it involves the same fundamental processes: raising a friendly eyebrow at glibness, and interposing a penetrating question into each comfortable elision of thought.

Clinical supervision at its best can be deeply disturbing because it leads to each of us being 'found out' – not in the trivial way we may fear, by exposing us as frauds, but in a much deeper sense. Supervision reminds us that we are partial and prejudiced human beings, who by preference will nearly always follow the mental and emotional paths we have trodden before, rather than daring to seek new ones. In that sense, giving supervision, and asking for it, may be one of the most truly scientific activities we ever undertake.

28 Welsh blood

I have Welsh blood in me. This may come as a surprise to anyone who knew my mother and father, who came from Vienna and Prague respectively, but I will explain the mystery soon.

My first visit to Wales took place in the 1950s, when I was a child of about ten. My father consulted the AA concerning the route to Snowdonia, as there were no motorways yet. We had to book phone calls in advance to the farmhouse where we were going to stay. It seemed at that time a place unimaginably remote from London, where we lived.

It turned out that the farmhouse, at the southern foot of the Carnedd mountains by Llyn Geirionydd, was even more remote than we had imagined. The road for the last three miles was unmetalled. It wound through dark forestry, past the looming ruins of lead mines, slate-coloured lakes, and a stark obelisk commemorating the great Welsh poet Taliesin. In the house itself there was no electricity, so we ate supper by the light of paraffin lamps and we made our way across the yard with candles – unless the fierce wind extinguished them – to the icy outhouses where we slept. In spite of the austerity, or perhaps because of it, we all fell in love with the house and the area. That love has never faded (although nowadays there is a pay-and-display car park by Llyn Geirionydd, a jetty for speedboats on the lake, and a 'heritage board' put up by the local council, giving historical details of the area for those in too much of a hurry to read a guidebook).

The farmhouse went through two changes of ownership, but on both occasions the new owners continued to take in holiday guests, and we continued to visit. In time, my father bought the former housekeeper's cottage a hundred yards up the lane. It became our second home and a family refuge. On two occasions it became a literal refuge, as relatives and friends emerged unexpectedly from eastern Europe and needed a roof over their heads. When my parents died we had to sell it, but my sister and I never stopped visiting that extraordinary part of Britain – both bleak and luminous at the same time – to share it with our own partners and children, and to visit local people we had now known for decades.

The people who now had the farmhouse became more reclusive and shut it down to visitors, but further down the road – past the tiny mediaeval church where Llewellyn the Great was married – another couple opened up two of their bedrooms to guests. So when I first took my wife up to north Wales, we began to stay there instead. It was an ancient long house, almost as old as the church, and formerly used as a lookout post for Gwydyr Castle in the Conwy Valley. There must be other parts of Britain where every corner breathes history and national identity like this, but I have never come to know any as well.

It was there that I was staying when I was taken ill. It was not my first serious illness, but it was possibly the most perilous, because the north Wales mountains are not the best place to have a gastrointestinal bleed. I went for a run to the lake and back, and when I rested afterwards, my tachycardia of 120 did not settle. It was then that I recalled how dark my stools had been that morning. Later a friend told me he had driven past in the opposite direction as I ran and had not recognized me, as I looked so ashen. That night, when I was already safely in a bed in Ysbyty Gwynedd in Bangor and on a drip, I virtually lost consciousness from a massive melaena.

It would be hard to do a controlled trial of the effects of landscape on hospital in-patients, but there can be few more recuperative views than the northern silhouette of the Snowdon range, as seen from the ward where I stayed. There was also something recuperative about the sound of the Welsh language, spoken by many of the hospital doctors and nurses as well as most of their patients. The sense of community and mutuality was strong, but I felt as welcome there as I ever did in the hills. When 'Songs of Praise' – recorded in a Welsh church – came up on the telly on Sunday, most of the men on the ward wanted to watch it, but with a tact that brought tears to my eyes, they sent a small delegation to my bed to ask if I minded, since they knew I could not understand Welsh, and was Jewish.

By then, of course, I was able to tell them how proud I was to have Welsh blood in me: six units of it.

29 Uniqueness and conformity

If you observe medical consultations closely, you will nearly always observe some kind of struggle going on between medical and lay styles of conversation. Patients mostly display a style that is best described as a narrative one, while doctors pursue one that is more normative. (The distinction is my own, but it closely follows the psychologist Jerome Bruner, who talks of 'narrative' and 'paradigmatic' modes of speech.)

Patients, by and large, have a story to tell. This story-telling has a primeval drive behind it, a drive that is universal and probably far older even than medicine. If you want to find out how powerful the story-telling drive is, you have only to interrupt patients prematurely in their narratives – as we all sometimes do – and to notice how they generally carry on from exactly where they stopped.

Doctors, by contrast, generally approach conversations with patients in quite a different way. Our utterances are largely aimed at matching patients' words against known patterns of description, or norms. These may be norms of diagnosis ('Is this angina?') but they may also be norms of degree ('How much has her breathing deteriorated at night?'), norms of behaviour ('Does she smoke?') or norms of treatability ('I wonder if this warrants a trial of an antispasmodic'). So while patients may try to carry on delineating the uniqueness of their experiences – and to take as much time as they need in order to do so – probably our own main concern is to find out the common denominators in these stories, and then to move our conversations to a close as rapidly as possible. Although patients are sometimes in a hurry and only want their doctors to get on with the task, and conversely doctors can be possessed by curiosity about someone's story and forget about time constraints, this discordance between the two styles is probably present during most of our encounters with patients.

Doctors seem to vary greatly in their awareness of this discordance. Some exert their professional power unthinkingly and as a matter of routine, ensuring that the normative style dominates every consultation. Effectively, they screen the patients' words for whatever corresponds to their own conceptual framework, ('blood', 'pain', 'smoking', 'pills') and conveniently tune out anything that does not. Most doctors are probably rather more tolerant of patients' narratives than this, at least in the opening part of the consultation, but they may still be waiting to pounce on any opportunity to bring the normative style into play, certainly as soon as they think it polite enough to do so.

One of the most difficult tasks in the whole of medicine may to be manage each consultation so that it continually meets both narrative and normative requirements. This goes far beyond so-called 'patient-centred' medicine. It means recognizing the equal legitimacy of the patient's need for self-expression *and* one's own need as a doctor to achieve pattern recognition, action and closure. It means finding ways to satisfy both needs at every moment in the consultation.

To do this effectively involves careful conversational micro-skills. In practical terms, the doctor has to try and interpolate normative questions or statements into the conversation only at moments that exactly fit in with the natural flow of the patient's story as well. Some doctors appear to do this intuitively. Others seem able to learn over time how to rearrange the strands of their conventional history-taking and advice-giving, so that these interweave seamlessly with the fabric of the patient's story. The most skilful can manage the conversations so well that they often achieve both normative and narrative closure at the same time.

In spite of the crucial importance of such conversational micro-skills, there is remarkably little teaching available for either medical students or doctors that is directly focused on developing these, and probably even less research on how some doctors manage to operate such micro-skills in practice. One outstanding exception is an article written by a team at Harvard Medical School.[1] The article includes transcripts from two contrasting consultations. In the first of these, the doctor does indeed seem able to pay attention to the patient's narrative in such a way as to find exactly the right cues for each normative question that needs to be asked. Here is an example:

> *Patient: ...my boss hadn't got all the parts for it, so I started working on another car, ya-know? That's when I ended up having the seizure.*
> *Doctor: Okay...So did your boss or someone else see the seizure happen?*

The doctor in the second consultation, by contrast, seems incapable of listening to anything except the deafening drumbeat of medical imperatives pounding inside his own head.

> *Patient: It's one spot right here. It's real sore. But then there's like pains in it. Ya-know how...I don't know what it is.*
> *Doctor: Okay...Fevers or chills?*
> *Patient: No*
> *Doctor: Okay. Have you been sick to your stomach, or anything like that?*
> *Patient: [Sniffles, crying] I don't know what's going on.*

Many of us will recognize an aspect of ourselves in the doctor's clumsy interventions. The patient's heartfelt exclamation – 'I don't know what's going on' – speaks to us poignantly as readers. What is going on is only too obvious. It is, of course, the institutionalized disqualification of the narrative.

1. Mishler E, Clark JA, Ingelfinger J, Simon P. The language of attentive patient care: a comparison of two medical interviews. *J Gen Int Med* 1989; **4**:325–35.

30   The refugee's tale

Valentina and Aferdita are both refugees from the former Yugoslavia who see me at the surgery. Their stories, on the face of it at least, are very different. (I have changed names and some other details here to preserve their anonymity.)

Valentina is of Serbian Christian origin and comes from Sarajevo. She married her Bosnian Muslim husband before such liaisons mattered very much to anyone there. Then, during the war, ethnic rage and murderous insanity possessed many of their former friends and neighbours. As a mixed couple, they were regarded as traitors by both 'sides', and so they left. Now, Valentina tells me that she would rather die than go back. She and her husband lack permission to work in Britain, so they sit at home for most of the time, fighting off apprehension and despair while they wait for their asylum applications to be processed. Understandably, they shun contact with their fellow refugees here. What keeps them going (just) is their infant daughter, born since they arrived in London. Valentina is also devoted to her studies, and now speaks fluent and expressive English.

Aferdita and her husband, by contrast, are both Muslims. Aferdita spends every minute of her life wishing that she was back home in her village. In four years in Britain, she has scarcely learned a word of English. A friend comes with her to the surgery every time to translate, and explains to me that Aferdita feels 'emptiness in her soul'. The friend knocks on her own chest to illustrate this. Aferdita also 'loses her mind' several times a day; the metaphor in this case does not seem trite, but evokes her loss of any bearings in her life. Aferdita grieves that her two elder sons have not seen their grandparents since they left their village, and that her younger son has never seen them at all. What keeps Aferdita in Britain, apparently, is her husband's passionate determination to win asylum status. If he can convince the authorities to let him stay, on the grounds that his life would be at risk if he returned, he will be able to earn a better living for his family than he could at home. Paradoxically, this would then allow the family, illicitly, to come and go between the two countries as they please.

It is tempting to see Valentina's story and Aferdita's in black and white terms, with Valentina's family cast as 'deserving' asylum seekers and Aferdita's as 'economic migrants' who could and perhaps should return home. However, I do not find such distinctions helpful. I wonder, for example, how far the stories that Valentina and Aferdita bring me have an aspect of performance to them – not in the sense that they are dishonest or manipulative, but because all narratives are told, to some degree, in the hope of affecting the hearer. Perhaps Valentina sees me as an ally in her fight with officialdom, and heightens certain elements of her story when we meet. By contrast, Aferdita's most pressing need is for compassion, so she too may be selective in what she says, hoping to draw me into an alliance that will further her own wish to return.

I wonder too how my reading of the two stories might change if I spoke with the two husbands – neither of whom I ever see. In the accounts I hear from their wives, both men seem to lack any ambivalence. Yet perhaps Valentina's husband is struggling with secret homesickness, or Aferdita's is too traumatized by the war to be willing to return – while neither man dares disclose such things to his wife. And if I could talk to some of their neighbours and acquaintances back home, who knows what frightening secrets I might learn, or new perspectives I might acquire?

Inevitably, I find myself thinking about the task faced by those who have to interview people like Valentina and Aferdita and their husbands, in order to make decisions about asylum. In this hall of mirrors, how on earth can they interpret what they are told? Through repetition and self-interest, even narratives that once bore a connection with some atrocious truth must degenerate into the quality of melodramatic fiction. Perhaps some immigration officers who have an unswerving commitment and adequate resources for investigation might sometimes be able to retrace the path all the way back from these stories to some historical facts. But common sense suggests that often this may not be the case – either because the path has become too murky, or because the commitment and resources are not there in the first place. The decisions that follow must be fairly arbitrary.

In suggesting this, I am making no claim for the moral high ground. These days, we sometimes spend up to a third of all our consultations in our surgery seeing refugees like Valentina and Aferdita. Such a proportion is common for many GP surgeries in London, and no doubt for some hospital departments too. We are bowed down by the workload, and without determined political action of one kind or another, it will become unsustainable. However the real dilemma for us, and for society, is that increased pressure on public services does not equate automatically with guilt in those who cause it – nor with total innocence either.

If we can contribute anything from our experience as doctors to the wider debate about refugees, it may be through avoiding the polarized banalities of politics and tabloid journalism, and by pointing out that the narratives told by refugees like Valentina and Aferdita are more complex, and harder to judge, than many people on either the political left or right might wish. When you are dealing with stories rather than visible scars, you cannot hope to eradicate abuses of the system, or injustices, let alone both.

31 Folk illness and medical models

Sometimes an author manages to capture the essence of an article with such an arresting name that you feel compelled to read it. A few years ago I was scanning a list of references when I came across a title so striking that I went to a library at once, to read through the article in question and see if it lived up to its promise. It was called: 'Hyper-Tension: a folk illness with a medical name'.[1] The author of the paper was the American social anthropologist Dan Blumhagen.

I was not disappointed. I now regard it as one of the most enlightening pieces of social science research that I have ever read. And although it is over a quarter of a century old – an aeon in terms of most academic writing – I still regularly use it as a set text when teaching groups of doctors and asking them to think about their patients' medical ideas, and their own.

Blumhagen reported on how he interviewed 117 men attending a hypertension clinic over a period of 12 months, in order to establish their beliefs about the condition. He found that each person appeared to have an individual model of what had caused their hypertension, together with a collection of ideas about how their body had reacted, and a further set of ideas about symptoms and risks. For example, in one typical individual the causes of hypertension included 'family arguments', the physical reaction was described as 'ballooning veins', the symptoms were felt as 'dizzy spells and flashing lights', and the patient feared the possibility of a ruptured blood vessel, leading to 'loss of a kidney'.

Blumhagen found that many of these individual models seemed to have a great deal in common, so that he was able to draw up a visual map of the 'folk illness', linking together fifty-seven concepts such as 'acute stress', 'narrowed blood vessels', 'heart attack' and so forth, with arrows of various thickness indicating the direction of causation as understood by a significant number of people.

No doctor who treats hypertension will be surprised by these findings, particularly the strong belief that the patients seemed to have in the psychosocial origins of the condition, and the even commoner belief that hypertension is symptomatic. But the real fascination of Blumhagen's work is in the discussion that surrounds these findings. It is impossible to do full justice to this here, but a few indications of the argument may give an impression of its richness.

Firstly, Blumhagen challenges the idea that 'folk' beliefs are entirely separate from 'formal' medical ones. He proposes instead that the two are closely interdependent, the popular condition of 'hyper-tension' clearly echoing the expert one, while at the same drawing on associations with more familiar words such as 'tension' and 'pressure'. He also demonstrates how individual illness beliefs are often inconsistent or may change rapidly. For instance, someone might describe 'stress' as a cause of their hypertension, yet later in the same conversation, when focussing on a different aspect of their experience, describe it as a consequence. As Blumhagen says, 'if one inquires about the physical causes of an illness, an explanatory model may be given which will be radically different from the explanatory model given by the same individual if one then asks about the spiritual or social causes of the same illness'.

In other words, what patients bring us when they talk about their illnesses is not some rigid and fully considered theory, but rather a loosely connected and fluctuating bundle of ideas, apprehensions and word associations, often oriented towards justifying a particular aspect of behaviour (for example, taking pills or not taking them, working hard or taking early retirement, and so on).

All of this certainly helps to make sense of what goes on in everyday consultations, not just with hypertension but with many other conditions. However, the main challenge that Blumhagen presents is to propose that the official medical model of hypertension may actually bear a great deal of resemblance to the folk version. He shows, for example, how the published medical literature presents a constant reworking of our professional models and belief systems, so that obsolete ideas slide imperceptibly out of view as if they had never been there, while new ones are written into the story in their place – each successive version being presented, of course, as ultimately authoritative.

Similarly, he demonstrates how different practitioners present their patients with versions of the 'facts' that are highly personal and selective in terms of what they include, omit or emphasize. Such explanations, although delivered with great professional conviction, mainly seem to serve the purpose of supporting the advice or treatment the doctor has already decided to give. These explanations also contain the same inconsistencies that you find with patients: for instance, a doctor might at one moment reassure someone that high blood pressure is unrelated to a stressful life style, while in the next breath offering the standard inane advice to 'try to relax more' or to 'avoid stress'.

Social scientists often tend to write about medicine in a way that can leave the ordinary jobbing doctor with a sense of futility and a wish to phone the pensions agency at the first opportunity, but surprisingly Blumhagen ends on a more positive note:

'Plain folk say "Hyper-Tension"; the experts say hypertension, and each thinks the other is talking about the same thing. Perhaps it is this muddying of the waters which allows both to function without cognitive dissonance becoming so great as to cut off interaction ... But there are occasions when dissonance caused by different models of illness does impede healing. At those times, a full understanding of the illness belief systems which are available to the layman and to the physician, if coupled with a willingness to negotiate a more functional set of explanatory models, may pave the way to a richer, deeper and above all more satisfying experience to healing'.

1. Blumhagen D. Hyper-Tension: a folk illness with a medical name. *Culture, Medicine and Psychiatry* 1980; **4**:197–227.

32   Minding the body

'You want me to see a physician?' The patient was clearly aghast. *'A physician?'*

Dr Barton sighed inwardly. He wondered, yet again, why the patients he saw in his psychiatric out-patient clinic so often found this suggestion unacceptable. The stigma attached to physical illness was still very great, in spite of all that the medical profession and the media had done to educate the public. Almost daily, he saw patients like this. They were only too happy to confess their deep-seated feelings of insecurity, or their unmanageable sexual desires. But they would nearly all conceal from him if, for example, they had had their gall bladders removed, or had ever taken painkillers. The sense of shame was too great.

'The fact is', Dr Barton explained patiently. 'We've investigated your symptoms very thoroughly. You've scored zero on the depression inventory. According to the interpersonal functioning scale, you're coping superbly. It's the same with all your other results. We really need to look at some other kind of explanation ... '

'But I don't understand. Surely you're not suggesting it's all in the body?'

It was a familiar response. As a psychiatrist, Dr Barton heard it almost every day. For each patient who was grateful to receive news of normal tests, there were ten whose faces dropped when they learned that they were mentally healthy. It seemed as if they placed all their hopes on being told they had something like manic depression or anorexia. They regarded the lack of a firm psychiatric diagnosis as a rejection. The implication that they might have a physical problem instead was seen as a positive insult.

It must be tough being a physician, he reflected. As a high flyer, he had never really considered internal medicine as a serious option in his own career. Indeed, his professor of psychiatry at medical school had warned him not to squander his talents on a backwater specialty like cardiology. A few of his friends had gone on to deal with bodily problems; they were strange folk on the whole, but you probably had to be strange if you wanted to spend your life mucking around with problems like blood pressure and breathlessness. He recognised that physicians did perfectly respectable work in their own way. He was just pleased he was doing something so much more prestigious and lucrative.

'Please don't misunderstand me', he continued to explain. 'I'm not questioning your symptoms. I certainly don't think you're making them up. It's just that we could waste a lot of your time doing more and more tests and still coming up with the same answer: you're basically sane.'

'So what exactly are you suggesting then?'

Dr Barton took a deep breath. 'Look, I'd really like you to see a colleague of mine called Dr Kreinschpindl ... '

'And with a name like that, I suppose he's a physician?'

'Well in a sense he is, but he's a special kind of physician, who tries to help people like you when we chaps can't find anything wrong mentally. He works with a team of colleagues from all sorts of fields: lab scientists, physiotherapists and so on. They nearly always come up with something. We call it our Pain Clinic.'

'But I keep telling you, I'm not in any pain.'

'Not consciously, no – but that's the whole problem. The body can work in strange ways. Sometimes people think they're miserable, when the real problem is that they've got pain all over. I've sent lots of people to our Pain Clinic and they've often been every bit as sceptical as you. They didn't think for one moment that their problem might be a rheumatic one, for example, or neurological. But once they see Dr Kreinschpindl they come away realising they were actually in tremendous physical discomfort. They've been very grateful.'

In private, Dr Barton actually had some reservations about Frank Kreinschpindl. He was a real oddball, even for a physician. His conviction that everything could be reduced to physical illness bordered on the fanatical. Yet, unusually for a physician, he had made a considerable name for himself in the academic world. He had published a ground-breaking study of a group of patients who were convinced they had borderline personality disorders, until Kreinschpindl showed that they all had nutritional deficiencies, multiple allergies or systemic candidiasis. His paper 'Toxic Megacolon masquerading as Obsessive-Compulsive Disorder' was also a classic. Kreinschpindl's clinical results were impressive too. Dr Barton would never forget a young woman he had seen who thought she was agoraphobic, until Kreinschpindl confined her to a wheelchair and put her on massive doses of steroids and immunosuppressants. She had never looked back since.

'Well, it doesn't sound as if you're giving me much choice. So how soon can I see this ... this physician?'

The patient spat out the last word with the usual mixture of fear and contempt. However, Dr Barton recognised it was a victory of sorts. At least he could now discharge the patient from his clinic, even if it turned out that Kreinschpindl could do little to help.

As he drew the consultation to a close, he began to wonder what the next patient would be like. With any luck, it would be someone with a more straightforward problem like paranoid delusions. He glanced at the clinic list and gave another sigh, but this time it was one of relief. He really was in luck. The next patient was a woman he knew well and always looked forward to seeing, someone he regarded as having real insight and integrity. And she suffered from the kind of problem that would inspire sympathy and commitment in any doctor: chronic somatization.

33 Escaping the loop

This is a story about intuition and its relation to logic.

A mother came to see me recently with her nine-year-old son, who wets his bed. She wanted me to write a letter to the council to support the family's application for a bigger flat. The boy apparently has two elder brothers who share his bedroom. They are fed up with the smell of his urine and want another bedroom.

When she made this request, I tensed up. I felt caught in a double bind. If I said no, I would probably lose any chance of helping the boy with his enuresis. If I said yes, I would effectively be offering an incentive for his behaviour.

Like most doctors when faced with this kind of dilemma, I found a solution intuitively. But afterwards I analysed what I had done and realized that it conformed rather well with formal logic and communication theory. This was a relief, as I was in the middle of preparing a seminar on this topic for a group of clinicians, and beginning to have my doubts about whether it fitted real life. I will tell you about my solution later, but let me go into a little bit of the theory first.

When Russell and Whitehead wrote their *Principia Mathematica* at the beginning of the last century, they proposed a Theory of Logical Types. A central argument of that theory was that a category 'cannot belong to itself'. To use the annoying language that philosophers love, the category of 'cats' is not itself a cat. More important, from the point of view of logic, the category of 'categories' is not itself a mere category. It is at a higher level of abstraction.

What this means in ordinary language is that categories of ideas or things have to nest inside each other like Russian dolls. They cannot ooze into each other like pseudopodia, or suddenly leap to another level like excited electrons. At first sight this may seem obvious or seriously uninteresting, but it matters in philosophy because it helps people to identify and disprove certain errors of logic.

A generation after Russell and Whitehead, the theory was taken up by the biologist Gregory Bateson. He suggested that logical typing is a natural as well as a mathematical phenomenon. He argued that mammals, including humans, seem to display in their communications an intuitive understanding of logical levels. They particularly show evidence of this in the ways that they respond to the same stimuli in different ways according to different contexts.

One example is the mock fighting that occurs among young animals. Cubs of many species can bite each other in ways that look just like real fights, but because they give out signals of a 'higher level of context' that this is only play, no-one gets hurt. If the signals about context get confused, no-one knows which is the higher one, fighting or playing. The situation then gets frightening and nasty. You can see this logical confusion when children of a certain age are practising their aggression but then lose control.

Another example is humour. Bateson argued that humour is often the consequence of an intentional confusion of context levels. We recognize this as a logical trick even though we may not quite understand how it works, and we find it amusing. (For instance, I once looked at a Japanese print of an elephant and commented that I didn't think that there were elephants in Japan. 'But this isn't a real elephant', the owner quipped. 'It's only a print of one!')

Bateson's ideas about logical typing in nature were taken up in their turn by communication theorists. They looked at conversations, and found that these tended to be harmonious if everyone shared the same assumptions about which context had the higher authority in any situation. However, things could become dysfunctional if this wasn't the case. So if one partner in a couple thinks that arguments are fine because there is an overarching commitment to work things out, while the other partner believes they define a relationship as a failing one, there will be trouble.

(On more mundane territory, most doctors will know of the discomfort they feel when patients respond to friendliness with intrusive personal inquiries. The patients are reacting to what they believe are the 'context markers' of an informal social situation. The doctors by contrast think that they are only being friendly as part of another, higher context – the courteous professional encounter – and they feel aggrieved.)

Returning now to my own difficult consultation, it is clear that there were two contexts vying for supremacy. One was '*the doctor as healer*' and the other was '*the doctor as patient's advocate.*' Whichever context I chose, I would automatically disqualify the other, and therefore fail in a legitimate part of my job. In communication theory, this is called a 'strange loop'.

Intuitively, I managed to get myself out of the loop. I said I was happy to write the letter but not yet. I wanted the boy first of all to attend the local enuresis clinic, and the family to make a serious attempt to engage with the treatment offered. If this failed, I would certainly back their application. The mother agreed at once. My guess is that the solution appealed to her in the context of '*the mother who wants a healthy child* '. She was now able to set this above the alternative context of '*the mother who wants better accommodation*' without having to let go of it altogether.

Of course the lure of better housing may lead the family in the end to sabotage any treatment, but I hope it will not. When there are strange loops around, disentangling them will often produce relief. Logic and intuition have converged. Could they possibly be the same thing anyway?

34 Dr Scrooge's casebook

'Dear Doctor,' I wrote to the medical registrar, *'This woman appears to have surgical emphysema extending from her chest into her neck and face ...'*

I saw the patient three days before Christmas. I had just completed my last surgery before going off for two weeks' break with my family. There was one home visit to do, then Christmas lunch with the team, and my work would be finished for the year.

I set off in the car to do the visit, but the Christmas traffic was backed up for nearly a mile, and I decided to turn round so as not to miss the lunch. No matter, I thought, I could do the visit on the way home when the traffic might be lighter. It sounded as though the patient only needed a quick eyeballing anyway.

I had already talked on the phone that morning to the domiciliary care manager who had asked for the visit. The patient was a woman in her sixties, a known alcoholic who lives alone and frequently has falls. The manager was concerned about an escalation in the drinking and the falls, with the woman apparently looking even more battered and bruised than normal as a result. However, the manager's main concern was that the patient's accommodation was clearly unsuitable. The neighbours were protesting about the loud drinking bouts, and they were afraid that she would injure herself. In the new year, the manager said, we would have to get the social workers in and get her moved to somewhere safer and more suitable. I noted the phrase 'in the new year' with relief. The patient was not one of mine anyway, so the long-term arrangements would be someone else's problem. I could nip in and out of the house, check that the woman was mobile and no more incoherent than usual, and still get home by mid-afternoon.

The traffic was no better at the second attempt. I cut up a couple of cars in order to gain a few seconds' advantage. When I rang the bell at the flat, the woman pulled aside the curtain in her bedroom, and signalled to me that she would come to the door and I should wait. She then managed to totter round to let me in, although she asked for my arm to lean on as we walked back to the bedroom. The place was bleak and disgusting, and I had to fight a feeling of being repelled by the woman herself. To save time, I asked her a few curt questions and checked her over while I did so. She had a swollen face that I assumed was the consequence of having two massive black eyes, but she managed to open both eyes when I asked her to. Her limbs were covered in bruises, and the skin had been sheared off her knees, with old slough in places. However, she told me she had made a cup of tea earlier and had drunk it. She also kept saying something about chicken and bacon, but I could not follow it. Her speech was honking and slurred, seemingly not just from the alcohol but perhaps from some other, lifelong impairment.

By now I was feeling impatient. I was angry about the traffic, angry about my vanishing afternoon, and angry with the colleague I was covering for (even though he had swapped the session at my request so I could get away). I had my own priorities, and making sense of the chicken and the bacon was not one of them – I wanted my holiday to start. Her condition was shocking, but no doubt chronically so. She was sufficiently mobile to survive, and to get to her phone or her front door. The care manager would visit again tomorrow in any case. I was reaching the point where I had decided to quit the flat and resume my life unimpeded by the needs of others, including people like this woman who live at the margins.

As an afterthought, I decided to check her chest. In the midst of the stuff about chicken and bacon she had mumbled something about being short of breath, but I had paid no attention, because I was only really concerned about her mobility. Now it occurred to me that she might have broken some ribs in a fall as well, so I reluctantly asked her to take off her blouse. As I pressed on her sides, I felt something I have only ever felt once before: a sensation similar to treading freshly fallen snow underfoot. Then I realised why her face was so swollen.

At first she refused to go into hospital. The chicken and bacon, it turned out, were going to be part of a lunch that she was looking forward to, and was still due to arrive from 'Meals on Wheels'. For various reasons, it took another hour to set up all the arrangements to get her admitted, including half a dozen phone calls and involving a further journey to the surgery and back to meet up with the care manager. The Christmas traffic was no better this time either.

As I finally composed the letter for the ambulance crew to take up to hospital with the patient, I reflected on how GPs manage to reduce turbulent experiences like this into the clipped, logical and efficient narrative of clinical medicine. How many hospital doctors, I wondered, would be interested in the larger narrative: the squalor in which we see so many of our patients live, the pressures that lead us to cut corners, and the guardian angel who looks us after when alienation and meanness of spirit threaten to take us over.

35 Yellow nose sign

A mother was describing to me how her child had been vomiting over the last few days. '*And I know just before he's going to be sick*' she told me '*because the sides of his nose turn yellow.*' She looked at me significantly, no doubt assuming that the yellow nose sign would mean something to me as a doctor and hence lead me to the exact diagnosis.

Patients' narratives are full of these kinds of apparently nonsensical descriptions. Mostly we do not even hear them – quite literally. If you want to confirm this, you have only to watch videos of your consultations. You will almost certainly find that there are details in every history, mostly about yellow noses and the like, of which you have no recollection at all. Because they do not fit the medical construction of the world, your brain either used the time to compute something more useful to you as a doctor, or deemed the details meaningless and therefore consigned them to amnesia.

As the sociologist P.M. Strong pointed out a long time ago, most people are caught in a double bind when they see doctors.[1] Often, their main reason for seeing us is precisely because they are not sure if they or their children's experiences fit the patterns of illness that we know about. Yet we get riled and suspicious if they trot out textbook accounts, and we react with selective inattention or mild contempt when they talk about things we do not understand, such as yellow noses.

Social scientists are trained to be more tolerant than doctors. They would take it for granted that the mother genuinely did see her son's nose go yellow each time that he was about to throw up. They would be untroubled by the fact that her notion of yellow did not correspond with my relatively inflexible medical concept of jaundice. They would also be vastly more curious about exploring the network of beliefs and explanations that enabled her to notice when noses turn yellow. They would, in other words, put her perceptions on a level playing field with mine.

What would happen if we as doctors did this too? One of the books that most influenced me as a medical undergraduate – as it did many other people at the time – was Thomas Kuhn's *The Structure of Scientific Revolutions*.[2] Kuhn argued against the positivistic, Popperian idea that advances in scientific theory came about as a result of systematic attempts to show falsifiability. Instead, he proposed a more sociological view. It was one that focused on how people in each generation develop perceptions of the world that do not fit with previous descriptions. Kuhn examined how people generally discount such perceptions at first, assuming that they must be distorted or incorrect because they do not fit with existing theory. Over time, however, more and more people share these perceptions, until they become the nodal points around which a new world view starts to coalesce. Once this happens, the old theory simple crumbles away. At first it becomes outmoded, then obsolete, and in time quite incomprehensible.

The best demonstration I know of this process in action appears in an essay about the history of asthma by another sociologist, J. Gabbay.[3] He goes through accounts of asthma from the 17th century to the 20th, noting how the shifts from one paradigm to the next are not small evolutionary ones but gigantic epistemological ones. Not only does the knowledge change with each version of asthma, but so does the fundamental nature of that knowledge.

Gabbay points out that it is tempting to assume that earlier descriptions of asthma will automatically map on to modern descriptions of asthma, or at the very least on to other recognizable conditions like congestive heart failure, pulmonary fibrosis, or even something a bit more remote like hepatic cirrhosis. Nothing, it seems, could be further from the truth. Seventeenth century asthma does not correspond in any way with modern asthma, but unfortunately it does not remotely correspond with anything else either. People with earlier models of asthma not only believed things we do not believe, but (as Gabbay illustrates in great detail) they saw things we cannot see, used treatments we cannot comprehend, noticed improvements we cannot credit, and offered explanations that are now impossible to follow. Each successive historical version of asthma consisted of a self-referential loop of symptoms, signs, diagnosis and treatment. None of its elements now makes sense to us, and none corresponds to anything that can be found in earlier or subsequent versions of asthma. The same, Gabbay strongly implies, will eventually be true of our 'asthma' too.

Doctors often find this kind of constructivist thinking hard to stomach. They believe that modern knowledge must be in some way entirely different from all previous types of knowledge. They find it hard to accept that even such fundamental notions as anatomy and evidence may one day be replaced by other constructions that we are incapable of even dreaming about. Many sociologists see this limitation in our thinking as simple defensiveness. They would argue that we are locked into our own mind sets by self-selection and then by professional indoctrination, We inevitably feel threatened by the idea that our whole system of scientific belief will one day dissolve and leave not a wrack behind. Yet if Gabbay is right, that dissolution is inevitable. And if Kuhn is right, the next medical paradigm may well depend on someone taking yellow noses seriously.

1. Strong PM. *The Ceremonial Order of the Clinic: parents, doctors and medical bureaucracies*. London, Routledge and Kegan Paul, 1979.
2. Kuhn T. *The Structure of Scientific Revolutions*. Chicago, University of Chicago, 1970.
3. Gabbay J. Asthma attacked? Tactics for the reconstruction of a disease concept. In: Wright T, Treacher A, eds. *The Problem of Medical Knowledge: examining the social construction of medicine*. Edinburgh, Edinburgh University Press, 1982.

36 The itch

I have just run the hot water tap and put my hands underneath it, with the water as hot as I could bear for as long as I could bear. The water was probably hotter than most people could stand, certainly beyond the temperature to cause pain. That was why I did it. I have been trying to reach the pain threshold in order to 'crack' the itch from my eczema.

To its sufferers, eczema is not principally a disease of appearance. It is a disease of itch. The itch is at times intolerable. Only hot water close to boiling point will crack it. Almost everyone with eczema knows this. It is part of the subjective knowledge that binds us: a knowledge that lies in a quite different dimension from anything you will ever read in text books.

I have had eczema all my life. It is hard to be certain how much of my disposition as an adult is due to eczema and how much to other parts of my inheritance from biology and biography. But it would be odd if it did not have its inner representations in habits of thought, feeling, images and relationships. From what I know of myself, I would say that eczema and the struggle to live with it earlier on in my life have shaped me to a significant degree. Perhaps this is true of everyone who has had significant illness in childhood.

Nowadays my eczema is limited to my hands and is entirely manageable, but as I child I had eczema in many places, including the inside of my elbows, behind my knees and around my ankles. Many of my memories of childhood are memories of disordered skin sensation: the itch itself, the incessant and futile struggles to resist it, the almost erotic release of surrendering to it, and the unbearable tension of trying to scratch enough to relieve the itch without gouging down to the flesh. Often, it was impossible to sustain the tension. I would give way to a frenzy of scratching, often privately in the toilet, where no-one could see what I was doing. The frenzy would lead in turn to other sensations: the immediate rawness of the newly weeping patches, followed in due course by the downright pain of hardened, stiffened and cracking skin. The rawness was usually accompanied by shame, the stiffness by a kind of despair.

I was born in the days before topical corticosteroids, so the memory of the condition itself is mixed with the pungent and sometimes brutal treatments that were in fashion at the time. My hands and much of my body were smothered nightly in coal tar ointment that got smeared all over my bedclothes and pyjamas. I had cotton gloves tied on to my hands in vain attempts to limit the damage from scratching, and at times my arms were put in cardboard tubes overnight to prevent me getting to my elbows. Later, I was taken to the old skin hospital in the west end of London for radium treatment, until this was found to be a good way of inducing leukaemia.

Like almost every other disease, eczema is an interactional condition as well as an intrinsic one. When my parents fought, which they did a great deal, I would itch and scratch more. My scratching and itching probably exacerbated their bad moods and sense of helplessness as well. Because of its shocking visibility, eczema is a social condition too. At primary school, the only girl I could dance with was one I did not much care for, who was herself afflicted with dry and scaly skin. She had no other choice of partner either. Oddly, I found her skin particularly repulsive because its appearance and texture was not the same as mine. I suspect now that she had ichthyosis.

At least the teachers in that school let me cover some of my worst patches with long trousers. When I started at secondary school, I shivered in grey flannel shorts while other boys stared at my legs and wondered (or so I thought) what terrible diseases they might catch from me. In the swimming pool and on the rugby field, I contrived to keep the backs of my legs out of people's sight lines as much as I could. Scratching, as always, still went on out of view. Probably very few people noticed the powdering of dry skin flakes on cubicle floors, and almost certainly they would not have known what to make of it.

A few years later on, I discovered how to use my understanding of eczema productively. While I was a medical student, I joined together with about fifty other sufferers and parents to establish the National Eczema Society. In time, I sat on its research and scientific committees, and I am now proud to be one of its first honorary life members. At a more mundane level, I also take pride in being able to explain the minutiae of skin care to eczematous patients or their parents. For example, I know how important it is to be meticulous about exactly how to apply emollients – on newly washed skin that is still slightly damp. I also know how pointless and infuriating it is to be told 'Don't scratch!' I sometimes advise parents to tell their children 'Don't itch!' If nothing else, the paradoxical injunction may stop them in their tracks and invite them to respect the compulsiveness of the condition.

The corollary of this knowledge is an awareness of how vast my ignorance must be of the subjective experience that lies behind all the diseases that I see but have never suffered from myself. At least that ignorance is a handicap I share with every other doctor.

37 Impaled on the invisible

Driving into work recently, I was listening to the 'Today' programme on the radio. Someone was talking about global warming, and quoting a statement from the Confederation of British Industry. 'Any measures taken to prevent global warming', went the statement, 'must not do any harm to British industry.' My ears pricked up. I wondered if anyone would challenge this tosh, but of course no-one did. Yet an intelligent ten-year-old could tell you that you cannot reduce global warming without harming industry. Conversely, if you do not take some measures that will harm industry, there will almost certainly be more global warming. That indeed is the dilemma.

Later the same day, I came across a similar argument. A friend asked me to look at an article he was writing about failed asylum seekers and the restrictions being placed on their use of the NHS in Britain. I read the article. It was passionate and polemical, but I doubted if it would convince anyone who was not already convinced. I asked my friend provocatively if he was proposing to open Britain and its health service to anyone in the world, regardless of their nationality or level of need. (He looked troubled for a moment. I don't normally ask such illiberal questions.) I pointed out that his article was similar to the statement I had heard on the radio. It involved the denial of a dilemma.

Denied dilemmas are incredibly common. Once you start noticing them, you spot them everywhere. Politics is almost entirely based on them. Every speech, every manifesto, is either for something or against it. Certainly, very few politicians – at least in public – seem able to frame any issue as a painful dilemma and to confess that they are proposing what they hope, on the balance of probabilities, to be the 'least worst' option. ('*My fellow Americans, we are going to fight a war. Perhaps it will lead to peace, and perhaps it will make things worse. We may be saving more lives, or putting more at risk. I simply ask you to back my hunch that on balance this is the right thing to do ...* ')

In theory at least, doctors are in a very different position from politicians. We are not obliged by our calling to take up postures where we deny the existence of dilemmas. Nor do we have to conceal any private doubts we may have, in order to stay in our jobs. In spite of this, I believe that we may not be any better at spotting dilemmas, or naming them, than politicians are.

One particularly fashionable way for doctors to deny dilemmas these days is for them to quote scientific evidence in a way that implies that it abolishes any possibility of a dilemma ('*Studies show that these pills will lower your chances of a heart attack*'). In fact, this habit is usually lazy, ignorant or disingenuous.

The more we acquire evidence, the more we should actually become aware of alternative options, and therefore of the need to offer complex choices to patients. (*'If you do 'x', these are the likely consequences. If you do 'y', these are the different consequences. Or you could do nothing and this is what might follow'.*) Contrary to what many doctors seem to believe, evidence-based medicine should lead us away from certainty, and closer to decisions that are based on patients' preferences, values and intuition – just as they always were.

I spend a fair amount of time doing clinical supervision and as I listen to the anxious narratives that doctors bring about cases that are upsetting them, I find denied dilemmas popping up all over the place. Often, the doctors who present cases have understood their problems in terms of conflict, but not as dilemmas. Asking people to reframe their problems as dilemmas can have a quite instant effect, sometimes with a visible jolt, as clarity replaces muddle. (*'If I declare this patient unfit for work I'm not being honest. But if I refuse, I may lose his co-operation'*) Often, such a reframing will lead to a resolution to hand the dilemma back fairly and squarely to where it belongs: with the patient.

From observation of doctors appearing in the mass media, it seems that members of our profession find it hard to admit that every medical issue has its dilemmas, however obvious the facts or the science may seem. The most solid of medical truths are embedded in provisionality, and ultimately we can never free ourselves from the dilemma posed by our lack of foreknowledge: *'This is what we doctors believe at the moment, but we have made asses of ourselves in the past, and we may be making asses of ourselves again ... '*

38 Fathers and sons

Oedipus, as everyone knows, inadvertently murdered his father and had sex with his mother. According to the story, he had not seen his parents since infancy, so he could not recognize the man he killed at the cross-roads, nor the queen whose city he saved from a plague, and whom he then married.

It is hard to know if people nowadays would be more familiar with this story than they are with any other Greek myth, had it not been for Freud. It was Freud – as everyone also knows – who believed that the story of Oedipus encapsulated a struggle that every child faces in its early years, as it tries to displace one parent in the sexual affections of the other.

Translated into evolutionary or neurodevelopmental terms, the Oedipus complex makes a lot of sense. It is a kind of deadly serious dress rehearsal for the later business of finding the best available mate, while remaining realistic about the scale of the competition and the limits of one's own sexual power. In some ways, however, it is odd that Freud placed so much emphasis on the murderous impulses of small children rather than those of their parents. In the Oedipus story, it is actually the hero's father Laius who sets the tragedy in motion, by believing a prediction that his son will one day kill him, and by issuing an order for the baby boy to be taken to the mountains and left there to die. The irony, of course, is that Oedipus survives to get his unwitting revenge – which fulfils the prophecy. In reality, parricides are vanishingly rare, whereas infanticides are sadly commonplace. It might be argued that we face a more precariously poised battle with our Laius complexes as adults than we ever did with our Oedipus complexes as children. Many parents would admit to having had to master feelings towards their offspring that were not far short of murderous at times. Even the most loving of parents will probably recall their first shocking awareness of being displaced by a ruthless, rebellious, self-willed infant with determined designs of its own – not on the marital bed, perhaps, but certainly directed at the subjugation of parental needs and ambitions.

If it is striking that Freud turned his attention to Oedipus rather than Laius, it is perhaps even odder that he did not concentrate on another story about a father with murderous intent towards his son: that of Abraham. It is a story with an altogether different outcome. Abraham, you will recall, follows a command from God to take his son, his only son whom he loves, to a place that God shows him, to sacrifice him there as a burnt offering. In a narrative of intolerable tension, we hear how Abraham takes his son up Mount Moriah, with a knife and wood for kindling, and binds him on an altar in order to butcher him. It is only at the last possible moment that an angel of the Lord stays Abraham's hand, and points to a ram caught in a thicket as a sacrifice instead. (In the biblical passage the angel calls out to him, but in Rembrandt's depiction of the scene, the angel seizes Abraham's wrist, thus forcing him to drop the knife out of his hand.) The angel then blesses Abraham as a reward for passing this test of his faith. The correct name for the story is 'the Binding of Isaac' but it is often referred to as 'the Sacrifice of Isaac.' The mistake may reflect many people's impression that Abraham's compliance with God's initial command is just as bad as if he had completed the act.

There are indeed many different ways of responding to the story. Many Jews, Christians and Muslims profess a straightforward admiration for Abraham's submission to God's will, regarding it either as exemplary in itself or because it demonstrates Abraham's utter trust that God will always do the right thing in the end. Most atheists, by contrast, are likely to see in the biblical text yet further proof of a vicious and arbitrary God who – if he existed – would deserve neither obedience nor respect. There is a subtler reading of the text than either of these. It was the reading favoured by some of the mediaeval commentators, who saw the resolution of the story as being implicit from the outset. This kind of symbolic understanding of stories, where time is collapsed and events are seen as synchronous rather than sequential, probably came more naturally to people before the Enlightenment than it does now. The nearest that we can get to such an understanding these days might be to say that the story is a narrative representation of ambivalence. In his heart, Abraham is torn between love for the son for whom he has always yearned, and his wish to destroy an heir who will one day supersede him. His struggle is both internal and external, with a God who is (to use theological language) both immanent and transcendent.

Many writers have understood that the story could have gone either way. There are ancient traditions that include the suggestion that Abraham really did slaughter Isaac. And in a more recent reconstruction of the story, the First World War poet Wilfred Owen described his own times in terms of an obdurate Abraham who had heard God's first, fatal command but then ignored its revocation:

Behold,
A ram, caught in a thicket by its horns;
Offer the Ram of Pride instead of him.
But the old man would not so, and slew his son.
And half the seed of Europe, one by one.

As Owen realized, the drama of Abraham's struggle is an individual one but also a collective, and indeed a universal one. The choice between behaving like Laius or like Abraham is not a foregone conclusion at any time, or for any of us.

39 The medics of Myddfai

I recently logged on to the web site of NICE, the National Institute for Clinical Excellence, in order to check their official guidelines for treating hypertension. I was delighted to see that they offer the option of reading these in either English or Cymraeg. The sceptics among you might snort at this choice, for who in Wales could possibly be interested in such guidelines and incapable of reading them in English? The question, of course, misses the point. The Cymraeg version is there not for utilitarian purposes. It is there in the cause of continuity.

There are no indigenous people left in Britain, but the Celtic peoples, including the Welsh, have the nearest claim to being aboriginals, having arrived from central Europe several centuries before the Romans. Seen through Welsh eyes, the rest of us are all relative newcomers, whether our forebears came as Angles, Vikings, Normans, Huguenots, Afro-Caribbeans, Ugandan Asians, or whatever. The survival of some of the Celtic languages on these islands through wave after wave of invasion and colonization over more than two millennia is historically quite remarkable. Waiting last weekend at the till of Safeway in Denbigh, I could hear more people speaking Cymraeg than English – a fact that would astonish most of my fellow Londoners, who could probably not even identify the language if they heard it being spoken.

Most modern Saesneg folk (equivalent to the Scots 'Sassenachs', or Saxons) are fairly ignorant of how much of our history in Britain is essentially that of the Celts, and of their interaction with successive conquerors and competitors. Yet in the Middle Ages, when Geoffrey Chaucer wrote about 'thise olde gentil Britouns' he did not mean the people we would now call the British. He meant the Celts. In Victorian times, George Borrow, a Norfolk vicar who taught himself Welsh and wrote the classic travelogue 'Wild Wales', still used the word Briton to mean the Welsh, as opposed to English people like himself. One of the things that he shared with the Welsh whom he met on his journey was a hatred of all things Norman, including castles, fashion and snobbery.

If as a profession we showed some interest in our Celtic past, more doctors living east of the river Severn might be aware of Britain's longest medical dynasty: Meddygon Myddfai, or the physicians of Myddfai in Carmarthenshire. They can be traced back to the early thirteenth century and their line continued in the village for over five hundred years until the last of them, John Jones, was buried there in 1739. The first recorded name among them was Rhiwallon Feddyg, physician to the local lord Rhys Gryg (Rhys the Hoarse or the

Stammerer). Rhiwallon was followed by his three sons Cadwgan, Gruffydd and Einon. Their recipes are described in a manuscript which has survived from the late fourteenth century in Jesus College, Oxford. These contain directions concerning the quantities and methods of preparation for the herbal ingredients – most unusual for European medicine at the time.

Modern research into the remedies – now being undertaken at the National Botanic Gardens in Wales – is proving a challenge. Not surprisingly, the terminology for plants and herbs has been inconsistent down the centuries. Inaccurate translations into English have also confused matters, and in addition, the botany of modern Myddfai does not appear to correspond with the mediaeval account. All the same, Welsh pharmaceutical researchers are now looking at native plants specified in the manuscript that contain compounds similar to tropical ones that have anti-HIV and anti-tumour properties. If that particular project fails, perhaps they may at least establish the exact methods by which the physicians of mediaeval Myddfai concocted some of their more mundane remedies: for toothache, piles and halitosis.

As with much mediaeval history, the stories of Meddygon Myddfai contain some credible facts mixed together with a great deal of fantastical legend. Rhiwallon is said to have been the son of 'the lady of Llyn-y-fan', one of three nymphs who arose together from the lake near Myddfai, as an apparition before a local farmer. 'After a little conversation with them,' according to one version of the story, 'he commanded sufficient courage to make proposals of marriage to one of them.' The following day the farmer passed the lady's first challenge: to distinguish her from her two identical sisters. He did so by noticing the pattern of strapping on her sandals (after she had wiggled her foot suggestively to make sure he noticed). In consequence, 'the lady engaged to live with him until such time as he would strike her three times without cause'.

Inevitably, this second challenge was one that he was bound to fail. The different accounts of the story vary in the details, including how many years it took before he delivered the three disastrous blows, how severe they were, and how many sons she bore him before this happened. One of the accounts describes how he merely touched her gently on the arm three times to remind her to fetch his horse, saying 'dos, dos, dos' ('go, go, go'). It was enough: she returned at once to the lake, taking with her the seven cows, two oxen and a bull that she had originally brought up from the waters as her dowry. But she did reappear, at least once more, to present her son Rhiwallon with a bag of medicines.

Alas, there is no word in any of the versions concerning whether or not her bag also contained any official treatment guidelines, in English or in Cymraeg.

40 Let's talk about sex

Do you ever find your patients sexually attractive? Have you ever been sexually aroused while seeing a patient? Have you ever prolonged a physical examination because you were enjoying the sight of someone's body? Have you ever had an enduring sexual fantasy about one of your patients? Have you at any time considered initiating a sexual relationship with a patient? Over the past year or so, I have become particularly interested in these questions. I have also become curious about why it seems impossible for most of us to discuss them.

In ten years as a GP trainer, for example, I can remember only having one conversation with a registrar about sexual feelings. He was seeing a patient who was becoming infatuated with him, and possibly vice versa too. I handled the matter rather awkwardly at the time: I was able to talk about the patient's feelings and what they might mean, but was too embarrassed to help the registrar to speak about his. Fortunately, it all ended well and safely. More recently, I have been running workshops for medical educators on supervision skills, and I have been struck by how even the most experienced groups and individuals will skirt round the subject of sexual feelings, or address them with coyness. This happens even when we are talking about cases where these feelings are patently present.

Why is it that we find it so hard to own up as doctors to our desires as sexual animals? One reason, I suspect, is that we are participants in a far wider social game of denial. Almost every newsagent and garage in the country sells sexually explicit magazines, while satellite TV offers dozens of channels showing nothing but sexual acts. You can find the contact details for sex workers in thousands of phone boxes and shop windows. (At the end of our nice suburban street, the grocery store displays a card advertising the services of a '22-year old model, for men and women, three minutes walk from here: sex £20'.) Yet in spite of this glaring evidence, most of us continue to speak as if masturbation, or paid sex with strangers, were aberrant activities, compared with the assumed norm of satisfied monogamy, with perhaps an affair now and again. There certainly seems to be no measured discussion in society at large about the difficulties of *managing* lust, and the pressures, disappointments and shame that are attendant upon so many people's attempts to do so.

In this respect, I have found conversations with gay friends enlightening. Because of their relatively marginalized status, it seems commoner for gays to share confessions with each other concerning the strength and unmanageability of their sexual urges, and to disclose the stratagems – successful or otherwise

– that they have tried out in order to satisfy these. Whether frenziedly promiscuous, celibate or loyal to one partner, they often seem to find it easier to talk to each other what they are feeling and doing, without the double standards or dissimulation that go on in much of the straight world.

I wonder if we could also learn lessons by thinking more calmly about paedophiles and our attitudes towards them. Being predominantly attracted to children is probably no more a conscious choice than being attracted to male or female adults: any kind of sexual orientation is programmed at an early age, whether by life experience or by biology. I suspect that many people with paedophile tendencies manage to sublimate them quite successfully into kindliness or intellectual friendships with children. (I believe that I had several teachers at school of whom this was true.) I have also known some highly responsible parents of both sexes who confessed to being aroused at times by the touch or smell of their own children. Yet there is a widespread belief that people with erotic feelings towards children are automatically evil, and can never manage to suppress these feelings. This conveniently gets the rest of us off the hook: it implies that 'we' do not really have any problems in managing our sexuality, whereas 'they' all do. And by holding on to this belief, we may be pushing some paedophiles further towards becoming abusers, since we damn them equally whether or not they enact their desires.

This confusion between desire and enactment may be what stops us talking about such matters more sensibly as doctors. The confusion seems to be more acute for male doctors, perhaps because arousal by itself is more clearly visible in males and therefore potentially more compromising. Yet we know that sexual desire can become heightened in many situations, including some medical ones such as deaths and disasters. Counsellors and therapists are used to treating such feelings as data – important information about what is going on in the room, and the kind of information that needs to be discussed frankly. The difficulty that we find as doctors in openly discussing our sexual feelings towards patients may lead to unnecessary shame among colleagues who are in fact behaving quite impeccably. It also blinds us to what is being done under our noses and in consultation rooms by a minority of colleagues who do actually molest or rape patients, as several notorious cases in Britain have shown.

Desire is not a crime. Sexual abuse – of children, patients or trainees – is. In the work I do with medical educators, I am now hoping to be a bit braver in naming sexual feelings and in creating a climate in which they can be discussed. I suspect that many of us are dealing at any one time with at least one patient (or colleague or junior) where it might be positively helpful to be able to discuss such issues maturely and in confidence. Personally, I doubt if there is a single doctor, of either sex or any sexual orientation, who could not give the answer yes to many or most of the questions at the beginning of this article – if he or she felt this could be done safely. If we were able to acknowledge more as doctors that we are physical beings who have physical feelings, and that we all face a moral struggle to manage these, it might in the end protect patients more than if we stay silent.

41   **Dialogue and diagnosis**

This is a story so typical of general practice that you could almost use it to help medical students decide whether or not they want to be GPs. (I have, as always, altered some details in order to make the person involved anonymous.) The patient is a woman in her late thirties, childless. The story began about two months ago, when I saw her with some peculiar neurological symptoms. I was vaguely aware that she had had a miscarriage about a year previously, but this was not at the front of my mind when I saw her: she normally sees another doctor in the practice anyway, and the presenting, acute symptoms were too worrying to think about anything else.

I called up the duty neurological registrar to describe the symptoms. He thought I was right to worry and offered an urgent out-patient appointment. He saw my patient a week later and was concerned enough to do some imaging. This turned out to be entirely normal. When he saw the patient a month afterwards to tell her the results, the symptoms had in any case changed. They had become far less specific and more suggestive of general muscular fatigue. He sent her back to me with a letter raising the possibility of a chronic fatigue syndrome and suggesting that I should send her to a rheumatologist or someone with a particular interest in such states.

So I saw her again and went back to square one. This time I got an entirely different story. The symptoms were now mainly aches and pains and exhaustion. She had more or less forgotten the numbness and parasthesiae that had brought her to me in the first place and caused such concern. (I wonder if they were amplified from the original consultation onwards as a result of seeing doctors, and then dispelled by the normal scans. We sometimes forget that we make our own contribution to the construction of symptoms.) When I asked her to date her problem, she told me this time that she had had them about a year – considerably longer that she had said at first. This timing took us back precisely to her miscarriage.

Miscarriage. Childlessness. Late thirties. Suddenly I knew that I was going to hear quite a different story from the clipped, clinical one that I had elicited and possibly promoted at our previous meeting. And indeed, an entirely new story now came to light. The miscarriage had been, in effect, a cruel caesura in her life. Until she had come to the doctor with heavy bleeding, she told me, she had never even dreamed she might be pregnant. By the time she knew that she was pregnant, it was already over. It was the only pregnancy of her entire life – a much longed-for one that she believed would never happen. But she had lost it before there had been any chance to celebrate her fertility for even one minute.

She began to cry, and then she told me more. Five years previously, when she was still in her mid-thirties, she had gone with her husband for some fertility tests. She was told she needed IVF, but in the same breath she was told she did not qualify for this unless she went private – which in no way could she afford. She described, word for word, the consultation with the gynaecologist. I have heard too many such stories to discount them as exaggerations or misunderstandings. The local 'rules' by which the gynaecologist had excluded her from treatment made no sense, in logic or humanity, but she and her husband clearly had neither the education nor the emotional resources to challenge them. They had walked out of the clinic, and never requested or even thought of a second opinion. When she had grieved her miscarriage a year ago, she had relived every minute of the earlier rebuff, and felt its injustice bitterly. She recognized the cruel pattern in both events: the tantalising possibility of parenthood, coupled instantly with its extinction. Her consequent numbness had not been neurological but existential.

It was clear that she did not have chronic fatigue syndrome, nor did she need to see a rheumatologist or fatigue specialist. What was evident was that she needed someone to ask for and tolerate a narrative that was entirely different from the one in which we all colluded, perhaps necessarily, the first time round. She also needed to tell someone who was capable of hearing both kinds of story – the biological and the biographical one – and who did not find it at all surprising that human beings live in both worlds at the same time, and may not know which of these worlds to talk about, in order that things might change.

I am sure that encounters like this also happen in hospital and psychiatric out-patient clinics. But as GPs we work permanently on the knife edge, as it were, between the diagnosis of illness and the interpretation of experience. I know few GPs who cannot tell of such transforming conversations on a weekly or even daily basis. And I wonder how on earth one could ever quantify the outcome of these entirely private and unique exchanges: the time, money and endless frustration that are saved when people are headed off from further referrals, further tests, and further futile 'treatments'; and the healing that starts when a story like this has been told.

42 Bigger picture, lighter touch

I am proud to have organised the first European conference on systemic family medicine, although I have to confess that this happened more or less by accident. I have a good friend in Finland, Pekka Larivaara, who is the only professor of systemic family medicine in Europe. Pekka wrote to ask if he could bring over some GPs to meet like-minded colleagues in Britain. I sent round a few emails to people who might be interested, and then decided it might be fun to invite some contacts in other countries too. They passed on the message, and the event started to gather momentum. When it finally arrived we had 70 people from seven countries, and enough offers to put on four symposia, eight workshops and three plenary talks. It certainly didn't seem too grandiose at that point to call it the first European conference on systemic family medicine, so we did.

Systemic family medicine, in case you are wondering, isn't a way of delivering primary care intravenously. It draws on skills and ideas from family therapy, and applies them to primary care. Systemic practitioners pay attention to the family, the team, the organization, and a range of other networks including social and cultural ones. They examine how these influence human problems and, more importantly, how they can be resources for resolving them. Systemic practitioners prefer to focus on three-dimensional processes rather than linear ones, so they are interested in patterns rather than facts, stories rather than diagnoses, and the creation of understanding rather than mere 'solutions'. Sometimes, this means working with a couple, family or group rather than just with one individual, or with more than one practitioner in the room at the same time.

Clinically, systemic approaches are helpful with many kinds of mental health problems, with 'grey area' conditions like chronic fatigue and fibromyalgia, with unexplained symptoms, and with frequent consulters. (There is good evidence, for example, that systemic consultations with married couples are more effective in depression than other forms of therapy or than drugs.) Some systemic GPs, like Pekka and myself, have dual training in family therapy and general practice. Others learn the approach mainly through experience. Not surprisingly, some of us are also involved in team development, supervision, interprofessional education and organizational consultancy.

In many ways it was fitting that the conference should have occurred in such an improvisatory way. After all, systemic practice is itself about letting things happen rather than making them happen: in other words, about 'trusting the system'. All systemic approaches depend on the notion that complex adaptive systems, including human ones, contain an inherent capacity to change, if encouraged and allowed to do so. Although there is a tremendous amount of theory to explain how this works (ranging from cybernetics and general system theory to linguistic philosophy and social constructionism) it is easier to convey this through metaphor. It helps, for example, if you can imagine that you are taking a small part in a vast collaborative dance ... or offering people a few sentences in a vast and as yet unwritten play with millions of other cast members who are offstage and invisible.

Some people, particularly those with an artistic or religious bent, seem to grasp such ideas instantly. Others struggle with them, because they seem so much at odds with all that medicine has taught them previously about single causes and predictable effects, and the importance of reaching 'the right answer'. Even sceptics become convinced, however, when they have learned some of the core techniques of systemic work: neutrality, curiosity, interactive questioning, how to develop hypotheses in the round, and how to tolerate multiple views of reality at the same time.

There is, of course, a question as to whether systemic family medicine can really 'exist' as a distinct approach. How can an approach that depends on exploring different ways of constructing the world be pinned down with a single description? How can something so elusive, provisional and evolutionary be captured by a single, unchanging term? There is also a big overlap between systemic practice and many other contemporary ways of thinking: these include patient-centred medicine, shared decision-making, narrative-based medicine and complexity. Some of the people who practise systemic family medicine don't actually want to identify it as such, for fear of seeming too exclusive. If we are to be truly systemic, we will certainly need to watch out for early signs of institutionalization, or a hardening of the philosophical arteries. And if we ever turn into another boring orthodoxy, and lose our capacity to improvise, we will need to reinvent ourselves as something else.

43 Diaspora and coincidence

The glories of ancient Sparta were inscribed in blood, not in poetry or art. The ruins that still exist are scanty, uninspiring, overgrown and little visited. The modern city too is a drab place, laid out on a grid. If you have travelled to Sparta in the hope of recapturing the magical experience of seeing Delphi, Olympia or Athens for the first time, you will be bitterly disappointed. But do not despair yet. A short bus journey will bring you to one of Europe's absolute marvels: the Byzantine city of Mystra. A thousand years after Sparta declined, Mystra was the jewel in the crown of Byzantine civilization. Eventually it became its capital, with a population that exceeded 40 000. When Constantinople fell to the Turks in 1453, Mystra held out for a further seven years. Its philosophers, scholars and monks then fled to Italy, where they formed an important part of that great wave of exiles who contributed to the renaissance of Western civilization. We owe Mystra more than we may ever know.

Mystra possesses all the colour and drama that Sparta lacks. As one guidebook describes it: 'Winding alleys lead through monumental gates, past mediaeval houses and palaces, and above all into a sequence of churches, several of which yield superb and radiant frescoes. The effect is of straying into a massive museum of architecture, painting and sculpture.' The site, too, is breathtaking. In contrast with the dusty Laconian plain just below, Mystra rises steeply up the wooded hillside. On a summer's day, and with adequate stops to admire the frescoes and to quench your thirst, it will take you a good three hours to get from the entrance to the summit. And it is only when you reach there, that you realize quite how spectacular a place this is – for rising far above you is Mount Taiyettos, the highest mountain in the Peloponnese. The exhausting, exhilarating walk so far has merely taken you to the foot of a minor buttress of the range. To get to the top of the mountain, you would need to continue through the forests and the distant mountain villages that have now come into sight, and past the sheer drops and exposed rock pinnacles. It would take you at least another seven hours.

Gazing upwards from Mystra on my first visit there, I felt no ambition to conquer Taiyettos. And yet I had a most peculiar fantasy. I felt intensely drawn to the distant white mountain villages. Not only that, but I wondered if I could ever buy a house in one of them and retire there. I dismissed this whimsical idea quickly from my mind and turned back; I had a ferry to catch to Crete in a couple of days. But when I returned to England, I read Patrick Leigh-Fermor's classic travelogue of the southern Peloponnese, entitled 'Mani'.¹ There I discovered that in one of those villages, Anavriti, there was an abiding legend that all the inhabitants were descended from Jews. Was it remotely imaginable that my unexpected moment of yearning to live in such a place had been prompted by some atavistic chord being struck with my own Jewish identity? Ridiculous, of course, but I did more reading all the same.

I found out that the legend of the Greek mountain Jews was not nearly as improbable as it seemed. Indeed, the Apocrypha records contacts between the Maccabeans and the Spartans that go back to the third century BC. Over a millennium later, there were Jews living in Sparta – although a monk named Nikon tried to have them expelled, in exchange for helping the inhabitants to overcome the plague. A Jewish quarter survived in Mystra itself after the Turkish conquest, only to be burned down later by the more brutal Venetians. Maybe the village of Anavriti had been founded by the survivors of one of these upheavals.

A few years passed before I found myself back in Mystra, this time accompanied by my wife. It was, of course, unthinkable to miss the chance of finally visiting Anavriti. Following local advice, we took a taxi from Mystra to a gravel mill in the countryside a few miles up the road, and asked someone there to show us the trail head. Rather untypically for Greece, the advice turned out to be entirely accurate and useful. Soon, we found ourselves climbing in glorious weather along a spectacular *kalderini* – an ancient cobbled donkey track that had borne Mycenaean traders across the mountains to the coast, hundreds of years even before Sparta was dreamed of, let alone Mystra. Two hours later, we reached Anavriti with a sense of triumph. We collapsed into a bar in the main street, and ordered some drinks in our minimal Greek. Having finally arrived here, how would we find out anything about the place or its history?

'*How ya doing?*' were the first words we heard. Evidently, we had no need to worry. An elderly man had sauntered over to our table, sat down, and begun to speak in perfect Brooklyn. Introducing himself as Louis (we never learned his Greek name) he explained that he was Anavritan, born and bred. Originally destined for a monastery, he had not found the idea much to his taste. Instead, he joined the Greek navy and ended up living in the USA for 45 years until he came back here to retire. When he was a child, he explained, there were 4200 inhabitants in Anavriti, including 400 schoolchildren. Nowadays, the population was made up largely of retired Greek Americans like himself – hence the wealthy-looking houses and renovated roofs we could see all around us. There were now only six children in the whole village, although they still employed a teacher to keep the school going.

Louis told us about his own family. We learned about his son, his Cuban daughter-in-law and his Spanish-speaking grandchildren. He described some of his chequered career in New York and Florida, which included an episode of smuggling diamonds from Ghana. Most people, on learning that my wife is a rabbi, are somewhat fazed at first. Not so Louis, who at one time had been in the catering business in New York. There, he had a male rabbi as a business partner, and had known many female rabbis as acquaintances. His company had catered for literally hundreds of large-scale bar mitzvahs. (*'They don't do them now like the old days!'* he lamented.) He addressed my wife as 'Rabbi' at every turn. And then, suddenly, he cracked a Jewish joke and broke into Yiddish – the language of mediaeval Germany, carried into Poland and Russia by Jewish exiles, and then, half a millennium later, into America, to be picked up by every New Yorker of whatever origin.

Was Anavriti itself really Jewish, we asked him. Yes, he replied, that's what the old people say. According to popular tradition, the village was founded by Jews around 500 AD. Later on everyone converted to orthodox Christianity, he said, but they were proud of their origins, and disappointed that the young people took no interest in the tradition. And yet, to tell the truth, I think we hardly cared very much ourselves by that moment who had founded Anavriti, or why. Sitting here, with the ironies and interconnections of a dozen civilizations echoing in our conversation and reverberating through the surrounding landscape, all that seemed to matter was the miracle of chance meetings and inexplicable coincidences, and the enduring beauty of Greece itself.

1. Leigh-Fermor P. *Mani: Travels in the Southern Peloponnese*. London, Penguin Books, 1984.

44 Careers advice

The idea of the career patient came to me out of the blue. I was listening to a case presentation, of a kind that is dismally familiar. The patient was evidently seeing six consultants in the local hospital and a further three in tertiary centres in London. He was on over twenty different kinds of medication, including six analgesics. In the past fortnight he had attended two out-patient departments, and had alarmed the doctors there sufficiently for both of them to have organized urgent CT scans of his head. His GP was fighting a hopeless battle to try and cut down his drugs, encourage all the doctors to communicate effectively with each other and with her, and reduce the financial impact of his behaviour on the National Health Service. As part of this battle, she had just insisted on seeing him on a weekly basis to 'get to grips with his case', as she put it. Needless to say, the patient was delighted with this proposal. It was at this point in the presentation that I found myself asking the GP why she felt compelled to disrupt this person's highly successful career as a patient. If he were a physicist or an economist, I suggested, his level of commitment to his life's work, and his degree of imagination and intelligence in pursuing it, might surely have earned him a Nobel prize.

I said this in jest, but it was a serious jest. I was hoping to liberate the GP from her futile mission to rescue the patient from something he clearly had no desire to be rescued from. I was also trying to debunk an unrealistic expectation that I might be able to propose something magical as an invited 'expert' with pretensions to knowing something about clinical supervision. In doing so, I was drawing on a well-established tradition of using paradoxical injunctions in the face of perverse systems and insoluble conundrums.[1] Yet the fact is, I genuinely thought it likely that the only feasible option here was damage limitation: not to the NHS budget, and certainly not to the patient, but just in terms of the GP's time, frustration and exhaustion.

Career patients, it seems to me, have most or all of the following characteristics. Firstly, they have a tantalizing mixture of indisputable physical pathology on the one hand, and a vast collection of far greyer and less convincing symptoms, signs and investigative findings on the other. Almost certainly, someone will have failed to diagnose something fairly obvious like hyperthyroidism early on in their careers, and they will apologetically slip this into their narratives so that every subsequent physician will be wary of leaving even the tiniest stone unturned. Although they may have had numerous operations, both necessary and pointless, they are quite unlike Munchhausen patients, since they remain intensely loyal to their doctors, especially those who have most conspicuously failed to improve any of their symptoms. Also, their problems usually accrue slowly and in geological layers, rather than appearing as sudden and dramatic eruptions.

Next, career patients usually have a finely tuned awareness of the workings of the health service. In particular, they have an intimate knowledge of its failings, and its tendencies towards fragmentation and dysfunctional communication. This gives them an ability to provoke, intensify and make a mockery out of the inability of most hospitals or local networks to join things up. Although the mockery is done through intuition and with apparent innocence rather than by brazen calculation, it succeeds in getting doctors to carry out absurd and improbable interventions (like two CT scans in a fortnight) in preference to picking up the phone and talking to each other.

There is a very large literature on various kinds of patients who in some ways overlap with career patients: frequent consulters, heavy service users, somatizers, 'fat file' patients, heartsink patients and so forth. Much of this literature purports to offer advice about how to work more productively with such people. Suggested tactics include: psychosocial inquiry, reattribution of symptoms to life events rather than physical causes, the involvement of relatives and carers in consultations, and reflecting on the doctor's own negative counter-transference. Although such advice can be helpful at times (although probably not as helpful as its proponents claim), it never seems to work with genuine career patients. Probably they have too much invested in their career to exchange it for an alternative one, however persuasively this is proposed. As for the idea that there may be a skilled psychologist or therapist somewhere who can permanently transform their understanding of themselves into a more compliant mode: I shall believe it when I see it.

The big question in dealing with career patients, I suspect, is whether it is possible to hold on to a genuine sense of respect for them, as opposed to using the label as an excuse for dismissal or contempt. One reason for respect is that they are not doing something meaningless. Quite the contrary, their pursuit of medical care fills their lives with purpose. They have an occupation that is just as absorbing as many far more respectable ones and may in fact be less of a drain on the public purse than some others, such as opera-singing. In any case, it is possible that we might end up paying even more for the social consequences of making them redundant. Their job exposes them to genuine risks, but so do many other jobs that we admire. However, the most important reason for respecting them is that their profession is in a complementary relationship with ours: they strive to sustain our existence as we do theirs. Like career patients, doctors too can be devoted to the search for simplistic answers to complex and unfathomable human problems. We are, in a sense, co-dependent.

In the end, the only way we may be able to have any impact on career patients is by accepting their right to pursue their life's work freely. Working on this principle, the GP who presented the case I described has now reduced his patient's regular appointments from weekly to bi-monthly intervals, and is issuing repeat prescriptions on demand, except where he feels he is putting himself at risk medico-legally. I sincerely doubt that his withdrawal from co-dependence will make things worse. It is just conceivable that it might make them better.

1. Selvini Palazzolli M, Boscolo L, Cecchin G, Prata G. *Paradox and Counterparadox: a new model in the therapy of the family in schizophrenic transaction*. New York, Jason Aronson, 1978

45 Mysteries of the male

Why do males exist? If you look at any standard biology textbook, you will probably read that the point of having males as well as females is to promote variation by the exchange of different mutations, and hence to increase the chances of species survival. Unfortunately, most evolutionary biologists stopped believing in this explanation over 20 years ago. From a reproductive point of view, no individual is interested in anything beyond donating genes to the next generation, while species survival happens more or less at random, according to the whims of climate and geology. You don't actually need sexes in order to mutate and produce variation. In any case, most mutations have no effect, or mainly deleterious ones. John Maynard Smith talks of 'the twofold cost of males'.[1] Firstly, it is incomprehensible that any female should want to chuck away half her genome. Secondly, the males of many species are useless at doing anything except sitting around, getting fat at the females' expense, and – in the words of Richard Dawkins – duffing up other males.[2] Among some animals, such as elephant seals, the vast majority die as wasteful, disappointed virgins.

Given the cost of males, it is perhaps not surprising that there are at least 40 species where the female kills the male during or after sex. In the case of the praying mantis, she literally bites his head off as part of foreplay, and he carries on in a delighted reflex of posthumous orgasm. Females of other species are equally imaginative: male scale insects have been demoted to microscopic excrescences on their females' legs, while female angler fish carry their mates on their backs as tiny dwarves. More pertinently, there are many effective ways of reproducing apart from sex as we understand it. These include simple division and gene exchange, which have served prokaryotes so well that they have produced the longest-enduring of all species on the planet, as well as comprising the greatest number of species, and probably constituting most of the biomass as well.

Among other organisms, alternative methods of reproduction include budding, hermaphroditism and isogamy (i.e. two individuals, not distinguished as males and females, combining their genes). There are asexual variants among all sorts of creatures, including jellyfish, dandelions, lichens and lizards. Of the creatures who do reproduce sexually, some species have two sexes, but others have three, or thirteen, or 10 000 if you are a fungus. Many species alternate between sexual and asexual reproduction, either on a regular basis or occasionally, as the circumstances require. Bdelloid rotifers – tiny invertebrates who live in drains and puddles – went off sex about 80 million years ago, and have cheerfully diversified into several hundred species since then, without regaining the inclination. Maynard Smith described them an 'an evolutionary scandal'.

The various current theories about why males evolved and still remain in existence are nicely set out in Matt Ridley's book *The Red Queen*.[3] They are also covered in Olivia Judson's racy and wonderfully informative book *Dr Tatiana's Sex Advice to All Creation*.[4] Different theories rejoice in names like Muller's ratchet, Kondrashov's hatchet, and the eponymous red queen of Ridley's book (named after the character in *Alice in Wonderland* who perpetually runs without getting very far because the landscape moves with her). This last theory seems to be the front runner at the moment. It is based on W.D. Hamilton's idea that sex is part of a continual race to outwit external pathogens. What is clear, however, is that the consensus that existed on this topic from Darwin until the 1980s has totally broken down. The purpose of males has instead become one of the biggest unanswered questions in science. My guess is that we will eventually come to understand fertilization by males in a similar way to how we now understand the appearance of ancient autonomous organisms such as mitochondria or chloroplasts in the eukaryotic cell.[5] In other words, we will see it as an evolutionary compromise poised half way between invasion and alliance, parasitism and symbiosis, or genetic rape and informed consent. There is already much evidence to show how females resist the process physiologically (for example by stripping male gametes of all extra-nuclear DNA) and how males try to control reproduction against their females' will (for example, by killing off competitor sperm or genetic material in the female genital tract, or alternatively killing the competitors and their offspring directly).

If the status of males in evolutionary terms is an equivocal one, the consequences of sexual dimorphism are not reassuring for males either. In a review of the evidence relating to human males, my colleague and mentor Sebastian Kraemer has set out the scale of the problem.[6] Throughout life, men are more vulnerable than women on most measures. This starts with the biological fragility of the male foetus, leading to 'a greater risk of death or damage from almost all the obstetric catastrophes that can happen before birth'. If they survive these catastrophes, boys then have a far greater susceptibility to developmental disorders than girls. These are magnified in turn by our cultural assumptions about masculinity, and by our low expectations of males. The toxic interaction of biological and social ingredients shows itself in far higher rates of suicide and deaths through violent crime. Males also do worse in (among other things) scholastic achievement, emotional literacy, alcoholism, substance abuse, circulatory disorders, diabetes, and of course in longevity. Kraemer looks at how male disadvantage is 'wired in' from infancy and persists to the grave, but he suggests that we shouldn't necessarily conclude that maleness is a genetic disorder. Instead, he argues, we should show more curiosity about the reasons for boys and men being so vulnerable, and should pay more attention to redressing this in child-rearing and in medicine.

It may be no coincidence that questions about the 'raison d'etre' for males, and concerns about their relative deficiencies, should have arisen at this point in history; enough of the relevant information behind them would probably have been available to an observer in Darwin's time. The recent appearance of these scientific preoccupations may well be the consequence of understandable male anxiety. In the last few generations of our species, female control over fertility has developed at a rate so phenomenal that it may justify comparison with the sudden emergence of male-female reproduction itself, around a thousand million years ago. In evolutionary terms, it has taken only the twinkling of an eye from the introduction of the vaginal diaphragm and the contraceptive pill in the middle of the last century, to the widespread use of frozen sperm and extracted eggs, and hence to the actualization of human oocyte cloning. Within the span of just one lifetime, women have advanced through several enormous stages of biological liberation and have reached the threshold of elective parthenogenesis.

Assuming that the minor technical problems of gene damage during cloning can soon be overcome, and that legal constraints will in time be removed – assumptions that seem reasonable by any standard – it is possible that the women of our species will soon have the overall choice of doing with very few men, or with none at all. If, in the meantime, they can prevent males from destroying any environment in which to survive, they might be forgiven if they choose to follow the path that has already been pioneered by the bdelloid rotifers. Attempts to understand maleness or to redress its difficulties will then become entirely academic.

1. Maynard Smith J. *The Evolution of Sex*. Cambridge, Cambridge University Press, 1978.
2. Dawkins R. *The Ancestor's Tale: a pilgrimage to the dawn of life*. London, Weidenfeld and Nicholson, 2004.
3. Ridley M. *The Red Queen: Sex and the evolution of human nature*. London, Viking, 1993.
4. Judson O. *Dr Tatiana's Sex Advice to All Creation: the definitive guide to the evolutionary biology of sex*. London, Chatto and Windus, 2002.
5. Lane N. *Power, Sex, Suicide: Mitochondria and the meaning of life*. Oxford, Oxford University Press, 2005.
6. Kraemer S. The fragile male. *Br Med J* 2000; **321**:1609–12. [Free Full Text]

46 Crusades and mirages

He was, without a doubt, the most powerful man in the Western world. His friends regarded him as courteous and moderate. His enemies saw him as 'a combination of Christian piety, xenophobia and imperialistic arrogance', in the words of one commentator. He was possessed by a passionate and single-minded determination: to end the ceaseless conflict in the Middle East once and for all. By doing so, he believed, he could not only bring peace to that region, but also extirpate the danger that Islamic fanaticism represented to innocent Westerners. To that end, he brought together an unprecedented multinational force, drawn from most of the Western nations, although not all. Some observers at least were sceptical, believing that he had ulterior motives for his campaign, or was launching it on a pretext, in order to consolidate his own authority and distract people from other conflicts nearer to home. Almost from the first, the vast military project was bedevilled by unforeseen scandals and setbacks, including appalling atrocities committed by some of the Western combatants. And although the invasion itself succeeded swiftly and conclusively, it was not long before some people were questioning the price that had been paid, as occupation of the Middle East led to a cycle of attrition that made the previous state of affairs seem pale by comparison.

The subject of the first paragraph is, of course, none other than Odo of Lagery, Pope Urban II, who on 27 November 1095 addressed a great crowd of believers in Clermont, calling upon them to take up arms and liberate Jerusalem. It was in many ways an improbable proposition. Europe was only just emerging from a long era of internal wars and realignments. Up to that moment, no-one in the West had seemed particularly exercised by the state of affairs in the Middle East. The enemies that Urban identified as his target were probably the wrong ones anyway; the real threat came from more fundamentalist and aggressive factions elsewhere in the Muslim world.[1] Yet Urban's proclamation of the First Crusade galvanized the West.

Within four years – an astonishingly brief period if you take into consideration the logistic capabilities of the early mediaeval age – the Western armies had occupied Jerusalem. As Raymond of Aguliers, chaplain to the count of Toulouse, noted with satisfaction: 'In all the streets and squares of the city, mounds of heads, hands and feet were to be seen ... what an apt punishment!' This prefigured much that was to follow. In the subsequent two and a half centuries, Jerusalem fell and was retaken many times, in a desperate and bewildering succession of intrigues, alliances, partitions, truces, betrayals and reverses of fortune. Most of this was accompanied by utter confusion and unspeakable carnage. Finally, after four further crusades, in an ultimate irony, the *combined* armies of the French barons and the Sultan of Damascus fell to an alliance of Turkish mercenaries and Egyptian slave warriors, the Mameluks, in 1243.

It is interesting to try and understand the mindset of a man like Urban II, and of the millions whom he inspired to engage in increasingly pointless acts of brutality against a distant enemy. The most obvious feature of this mindset is what psychologists call splitting: an inability to see anything except virtuous motives on one's own side and malignity on the part of the other. The most atrocious deeds were perpetrated in the fixed belief that the enemy's misdeeds were sufficient to merit such punishment. War was seen as a necessity for bringing about peace. Indeed, it was accepted more or less without question that the best way of promoting a universal doctrine of peace was by imposing it through extreme violence.[2] This allowed the crusaders to see themselves as virtuous, even when it was clear that they were driven by economic motives and the raw pursuit of power. For example, from time to time they abandoned their own allies and turned to slaughtering them instead, including innumerable Greek Orthodox Christians as well as Jews. During all of this, they were able to sustain an image of themselves as noble and chivalrous knights, rather than as fanatical, avaricious, treacherous and bloodthirsty thugs, which is how they were generally seen outside the West.

Throughout the period, the crusaders therefore managed to maintain a fantasy that the very next campaign would end the conflict for all time. They were incapable of looking back at the errors of their predecessors or foreseeing the catastrophes that would follow a repetition. Hardly anyone understood that messy stand-offs are often the best that can be achieved in human affairs, or that a compromise may allow a population to live in a more tolerable state than interminable war. Two honourable exceptions in this respect were Frederick of Hofenstaten and Al-Kamil. These basically irreligious leaders managed to achieve a historic partition of Jerusalem in 1229, allowing free access to pilgrims of all religions. This was a similar state of affairs to the one that had existed anyway before the crusades began. They were both reviled by their contemporaries. Their treaty lasted only ten years.

The spirit of the crusading enterprise infused the whole of Western society. Many British place names still carry echoes of the barracks, banks, hospitals, estates and other institutions that supported and housed the crusading knights. Temple station on the London Underground and Ysbyty Ifan – St John's Hospital – in north Wales are two among many examples. The crusading armies were financed by the taxes, rents and donations of many of the Western nations. Essentially, whole European populations were implicated in the crusades, not least through their acquiescence in the idea that their civilization was superior to that of others. They tolerated the news of collateral suffering inflicted in their name on innocent bystanders elsewhere. They remained incapable of understanding that they might be seen exactly as they saw others, and were actually provoking complementary acts of barbarism. The only question the crusaders ever asked was 'what retribution should follow the enemy's crimes?'. No-one ever considered the alternative question: 'what retribution might follow our response?'

Our children or grandchildren may live to see the day in 2095 that marks a millennium since Pope Urban initiated this long era of mass ideological psychosis. Let us hope that they will inherit a world that has risen above such simplistic thinking, and such militaristic folly.

1. Read PP. *The Templars.* London, Weidenfeld and Nicholson, 1999.
2. Housely N. *The Crusaders.* Stroud, Tempus, 2002.

47 Weasel words

Here is a conference advertisement from a national newspaper:

'Choice Partnership presents Managing Care Services Improvement: a two day conference exploring citizenship, new realities, and sharing risk through promoting integrated delivery of health, housing and social services.'

Fascinated by the language, I decided I would put some of the phrases on cards, shuffle them, ask my wife to pick up cards at random, and then put the resulting sequence of phrases back into the original framework. We did the exercise three times. This is what we came up with:

A. 'New Realities Partnership presents Managing Choice: a two day conference exploring care services improvement, health, housing and social care services, and promoting sharing risk through integrated delivery of citizenship.'

B. 'Care Services Improvement Partnership presents Managing New Realities: a two day conference exploring choice, sharing risk and promoting citizenship through integrated delivery of health, housing and social care services.'

C. 'Sharing Risk Partnership presents Managing Health, Housing and Social Care Services: a two day conference exploring new realities, care services improvement, and promoting choice through integrated delivery of citizenship.'

Now I have to confess I have played a little trick on you. The original advertisement was actually not the one in the first paragraph but version B ... or possibly C, or maybe A. Can you guess which one? Of course not. Because the genuine version is just as vacuous as the scrambled ones. They are all equally devoid of meaning, a kind of political pornography, designed to induce a satisfied glow of righteous recognition in the same way that a photo of two breasts or a bottom is calculated to produce a different kind of glow.

Why do we not scream with outrage at the constant assault we now suffer from this kind of language in the public services? Or even better, why do we not laugh at it till the tears stream down our cheeks? I recently spent a morning in the presence of a score of senior colleagues while we all struggled with the question set for us by a highly paid facilitator: how were we going to rise to the challenge of consumer choice, a patient-led service, an accelerated pace of change coupled with necessary efficiency savings ... ? We all sat there like well-behaved children at an old-fashioned preparatory school, listening to this rubbish as if it meant anything. By the end of the morning we were actually *speaking* the stuff, as if we believed it, as if it had become part of us. Grown men and women, each with decades of serious professional experience, were jumping up energetically to add empty resolutions to the bullet points on two flip charts, under the fatuous headings of 'quick wins' and 'smart objectives'. For goodness' sake, what is happening to us? Can anything be done to prevent us losing our souls entirely to this fraudulent drivel?

Before I decline into permanent acquiescence with it, let me spell out some truths that may help us resist this pervasive deceit in the public services: (1) There is a close relationship between corruption of language, corruption of thought, and corruption of action. There may be some ways in which parts of the public services are improving, and it is even possible that some organizational changes are for the better. However, celebrating any patchy successes in increasingly messianic slogans leads to the disablement of any serious analysis, then to the denial of any error or failure, and then to systematic cover-up and abuse. (2) It did not used to be like this. There was a time in the recent past when people in the West read such bombast with horror, because we thought it belonged to totalitarian states where people were unable to protest at the blatant hypocrisy that surrounded them. (3) The practice of medicine is not a state activity, and doctors who are over-identified with the state, or with the language of the state, have sold out. Medicine is generally conservative and respectful of those in power, and it probably needs to be. But there are also times when medicine has to be subversive. Doctors who cannot act, think and speak subversively can be dangerous.

Thank goodness, we still live in a society where we can at least make fun of people in positions of power who tell lies to themselves or others, who take themselves too seriously, or who talk nonsense. We should take every opportunity to do so. As most of the population of Europe discovered during the twentieth century, it is a right that is quickly and easily removed, and then only recovered at an appalling cost.

48 The enduring asylum

'Loonies', they shouted from the back of the coach. 'Loonies!' I can't remember if we had reached the gates of the mental hospital yet, but I was excruciatingly embarrassed, and I prayed that they would stop. It didn't help me very much that I understood, to an extent, what had provoked some of the students in my year to such cruel mockery. It was 1974. Sociology had just become a compulsory subject at our medical school in London. The young sociology lecturers had arrived with a mission to radicalize the next generation of doctors, offering us the latest critiques of medicine and of psychiatry. An instructive coach trip into the countryside, to visit one of the vast Victorian 'bins' that still peppered Hertfordshire, Essex and Surrey, was not proving to be helpful.

In retrospect, we were all caught up in a painful historical drama concerning views of madness. The sociologists were fired with a conviction that everything we were about to see was a demonstration of how society oppressed and imprisoned free spirits in the name of medical treatment. The students felt provoked by this, and were no doubt fearful as well, and they regressed into viciousness. While our tour leaders looked forward to a Utopia in which schizophrenics would all be revealed as artists and mystics, the young men on the back seat were imitating the visitors who went to gawp and jeer at the inmates of Bedlam three centuries earlier.

I remember little of the rest of the visit. It is possible that the lecturers cut it short in order to pre-empt a scandal. But I do remember a visit some time later to a rural asylum for the mentally handicapped, where dozens of adult men just sat in chairs and rocked, or wandered aimlessly around the room, in a way that seemed more like a parody of imbecility than a demonstration of it. Then, during my clinical years, I was sent for about four weeks to study at another, different 'bin' for the mentally ill. Politicians had already decided to shut down all the psychiatric hospitals, but at this stage most of them were still much the same as a century before.

In the place I was assigned to, the corridors were allegedly the longest in Europe. On some of the chronic wards, scores of elderly women sat quite passively, staring into the air; it was said that some of them had been admitted decades earlier for having had illegitimate children. In the acute wards, one could still encounter the 'classic' cases described in the text books: people with agitated depression wringing their hands all day long, patients in a state of catatonia sitting like pale statues cemented into place, and psychotic individuals babbling 'word salad'. A hundred years after Charcot's clinical demonstrations, and more than a decade after R.D. Laing's scathing exposure of such spectacles, ward rounds still consisted of patients appearing every week or two in front of a panel of doctors and psychiatric nurses to 'display' their pathology.

It is now more than a generation later. These memories have been stirred up by attending a coffee morning in Denbigh, to mark the launch of a history of the North Wales Hospital.[1] Like the great asylums around London, the hospital once housed 1500 mental patients and employed around 1000 staff. Since its closure in 1995, the grand buildings have stood empty, decaying quietly while developers and councils wrangle over its future. The town's identity has been stamped with its ambiguous inheritance as a centre of care and of incarceration. In some ways it is still waiting to find a new purpose as a community, while these wrangles are resolved.

At the book launch, two former psychiatric nurses from the hospital (one now a historian, and author of the book) mourn the passing of the institution, but with no illusions or regrets. They are reconciled to the harm that it did, both to its inmates and to themselves. Now in retirement, they work for voluntary organizations, visiting some of the people who were discharged from the wards into homes around the town, and making sure that their everyday needs are being met. Ironically, they explain how they now feel discounted as mere volunteers by the professionals who populate the brave new world of community mental health care. For example, psychiatric reports are written with no mention of their work with patients, or the social activities they lay on to keep these people's minds alive.

Listening to them, I am reminded of how we still remain in thrall to the asylum mentality. The asylums of brick and stone, thank God, have now been closed down; we have learned to acknowledge that the madness we observed there was largely manufactured by the institutions themselves, rather than in the minds of their inhabitants. But the virtual asylums have endured. As the two nurses have discovered, we remain in a state of mind where professionals can still ignore any involvement from lay carers. There is also the mental health 'team', where anonymity and bureaucracy stand in place of iron gates and locked wards. We construct another asylum out of the self-important distinctions by which a dozen different mental health professions and theoretical camps insist on identifying themselves, and bewildering everyone else. Finally, there are the tick-box inventories by which we try to pretend that mental distress can be reduced to the same kind of diagnostic categories as TB or appendicitis, and entirely divorced from any social or cultural context.

The foolish boys shouting 'Loonies' on the bus to Shenley could never have dreamed that the whole site would one day be converted into luxury homes for City commuters and the rural rich, as it is now. I hope that today's medical students will see a day when our own virtual asylums vanish, and are replaced in their turn by more humane care.

1. Wynne C. *The North Wales Hospital, Denbigh 1842–1995/Ysbyty Gogledd Cymru, Dinbych 1842–1995* 2006; Rhyl Gwasg Heligain, 2006.

49 Do not disturb

The waiting room was clean and tidy but rather drab, and lacking in any friendly touches like paintings or historical photos. What particularly caught my attention were the notices on the walls and around the reception desk. 'Don't consume food and drink, or chew gum in the waiting room.' 'Don't ask the doctors for housing letters as we do not issue them.' 'Unused drugs cost the NHS £5.2 billion pounds a year' (how does anyone know, I wondered) 'so don't ask for items that you don't really need'. 'Remember that appointment slots are only for ten minutes. Don't compromise your care by asking the doctor to deal with more than one problem.' Altogether, I counted eleven 'don'ts', and not one 'please'.

I was only there to interview one of the doctors, not as a patient, but I felt quite desolate nonetheless. I pondered on the peculiar idea that medical problems should all be presented singly. Would you be allowed to mention, for example, that you had both chest pain *and* shortness of breath? If you were worried about a sore throat, would the worry disqualify you from mentioning the throat, or possibly vice versa? I recalled a patient I once saw who came in and said: 'I've got three problems'. Acting on an intuition, I asked her: 'What's the fourth?' She told me. It was the problem that she both dreaded and desperately wanted to tell me, and we never got back to the original three problems. I considered telling this anecdote to the doctor once he called me through, and perhaps to talk a little about making space for narratives in medicine as well as numbers. But I was here to conduct research, not to deliver a homily, so I dismissed the idea from my mind.

A receptionist led me upstairs. This was clearly not a doctor used to coming to greet colleagues, let alone patients. He did at least stand up to shake my hand: a smart, pleasant, efficient-looking young man. After some social niceties, I took him through the preliminary part of the interview, which addressed various ethical dilemmas that GPs face in their everyday work. He was thoughtful about them, to a degree, but took little time to reach a clear conclusion on each. Every time he did so, there was a distinct tone of finality in his voice. I had no difficulty imagining what it would be like to be a patient of his. If my blood pressure was high, for example, every ounce of his authority would be harnessed to persuading me to swallow the optimal medication. But if I wanted to speak of matters of the heart, or of the soul, I would have no expectation of being heard, and would keep them to myself.

As part of the research, I asked him if he could give me an example of one recent ethical dilemma that he had handled well, and another where he had doubts about what he had done. In response, he mentioned two encounters that he felt had both gone rather well. In the first, he had to explain to a childless woman of forty that there was no funding available locally for someone of her age to have IVF. The second patient was a community nurse, a few years away from retirement, who was seeing him regularly with minor illnesses in order to request sick certificates. He seemed proud of having told her the previous day that enough was enough, and she should now return to work. He told these stories in a clipped, peremptory manner. I did not get any impression that he had tried to engage with the painful existential struggles that presumably lay under the surface of these requests.

Because the protocol of the interview allowed me to do so, I mentioned to him that he seemed unperturbed, and possibly imperturbable, by any of these dilemmas. I took the risk of asking him what perturbed him in his everyday life outside medicine. To do him justice, he blushed slightly and told me about an incident when he got angry with one of his children. But when I asked if such anger ever played a part in his consultations, he looked perplexed, and I knew I could not go there.

Doctors like this have a strange effect on me. I start to become anxious that my pre-occupation as an educator with such things as dilemmas, narratives, feelings, ethics, complexity, meaning and (God help me) consultation skills, is really just a projection of my own tortured psyche. Maybe if my upbringing had not been troubled, or if I had not had any therapy, or trained as a therapist, I would see the world in its true light, just as this man sees it: in terms of right and wrong, black and white, and problems that come only in the singular and never in the plural. I begin to wonder if I really am a doctor, or if I have ever been one. I certainly feel at moments like this that I have never been a very skilled or knowledgeable one. Perhaps I have just muddled through in a fog of doubts and uncertainty, never actually making anyone better – unless this was going to happen to them anyway.

In this state of mind, I closed the interview and made my exit, but as soon as I was back in the waiting room I saw all those 'Don'ts' again and my sense of self returned. So too did my sense of the impoverishment of this man's experience of medicine. For what notices like this in waiting rooms really proclaim is this: 'We are afraid. Afraid of intimacy, afraid of suffering, afraid of everything we do not understand and cannot cure.' And the missing 'pleases' are all too clear as well: 'Please remember that you are here to make us feel good, not the other way around. Please do not challenge us because, in reality, we are too vulnerable to cope.'

50 **Burning your relatives**

If you want to dispose of a dead body, either human or animal, there are only a few ways you can do it, and they all have much the same effect. You can leave the body out in the open, so that other creatures of various kinds can eat most of it, metabolizing it into water and carbon dioxide. The bits that remain will be oxidized, essentially undergoing the same process but more slowly. An alternative option is to burn the body. This will also lead to the same results, but of course at a much faster rate. Or you can slow the process down by burying the body in the earth or at sea. In that case, consumption of the body by other creatures may still take place, but oxidization of the uneaten remains will not occur until the body is somehow exposed to the atmosphere once more.

In certain circumstances, geological change on top of a burial site will compress bodies and reposition them at increasing depths under the surface of the earth; in the case of some species – marine animals are a case in point – they may remain there for considerable periods of time, perhaps even millions of years. If you eventually disinter such long-buried corpses in the form of their liquefied or gaseous residues, you can ignite them with a spark in an enclosed space, and produce a very accelerated form of combustion, thereby releasing great amounts of energy. This process was perfected around 150 years ago, when Etienne Lenoir invented the internal combustion engine. Since then, we have been burning dead plankton at a tremendous pace. At a rough estimate, reserves of marine corpses took about a hundred million years to build up (although in reality this probably took place only in short epochs during that time). We have probably got through over half of these reserves already, and at the present rate of usage, the rest is unlikely to last us another forty years. Currently we are burning dead marine animals at around a million times the rate that it took to create them. This is comparable to raising a fellow human being for 25 years, and then burning him or her up for fuel purposes alone in around a minute.

There are a number of peculiarities about this business. One is that we are undoing a planetary process that has allowed us to emerge as a species, and to survive. If every organism remained on the surface of the earth after death, decomposition would soon replace much of the oxygen in the atmosphere with carbon dioxide. This would possibly reduce the net balance of surviving animals to nil. It is only the accidental burial of a large proportion of creatures that has sustained enough free oxygen to result in our own existence, and we are now reversing that process. Another peculiarity is our emotional disengagement from what is happening. Even if we are aware of the fact intellectually, we do not as a rule drive around in our cars exclaiming: 'Oh my God, I am cremating my ancestors and cousins in prodigious quantities, and turning them into noxious gases!' But that of course is exactly what we are doing.

It has become fashionable recently to try and become aware of some of the damage that we are doing by burning our fossils, not because we are worried about oxygen depletion in the very long term but because it will warm up the globe in the very short term. There are now schemes that allow you to calculate how much carbon dioxide you are putting into the atmosphere personally, mainly through the means of transport that you use, and to 'pay it back' symbolically by funding the planting of trees. These schemes are based on units of carbon consumption per year, although an alternative approach would be to look instead at the time it took to create the fuel we consume, and to compare this with the time it takes us individually to burn it up. It seems that the planet produced around 380 thousand billion litres of oil in total; according to this estimate, a three-hour car trip up the motorway using 38 litres of petrol will consume roughly the amount that it would have taken the entire earth five minutes to produce. On this basis, it should be fairly easy to work out how many 'earth hours' of fossil production you use up each year by car travel. (I have obtained all the figures here from the internet and done the sums on the back of the proverbial envelope, since I cannot find these calculations anywhere else. If anyone is inspired to work out a more scholarly formula, I will be very pleased. Even if my arithmetic is wrong, I doubt that the result will be reassuring.)

One irony about this rate of oil consumption is that we are using the stuff up so fast that it may run out before the effects of its combustion become terminal. Economists and politicians tend to speak out either about global warming, or about the exhaustion of oil supplies, but they rarely address both at the same time. Yet the real challenges that face the world are likely to be due to the social and political consequences of a coincidental interplay between these two processes. There is no logical reason in evolutionary history why global warming should not have happened long before we were able to use up all the oil, or vice versa, and it is tempting to imagine some unfathomable meaning in the fact that these are more or less going to converge. The ancient prophets of many religions may have used expressions that we now find alienating, when they made a connection between impending natural calamities and our failings as human beings. They may also have been slightly awry in their predictions about the timing. But intuitively they understood the fundamental nature of the problem: we think as individuals and with our heads, but we cannot act collectively and with our hearts.